FASTING

2-IN-1 BUNDLE

This book includes:

Intermittent Fasting & Bodybuilding

Intermittent Fasting

Lose Fat, Build Muscle, and Get Fit

Table of Contents

hardship or damages that may befall them after undertaking information described herein.

Additionally, the information found on the following pages is intended for informational purposes only and should thus be considered, universal.

As befitting its nature, the information presented is without assurance regarding its continued validity or interim quality.

Trademarks that mentioned are done without written consent and can in no way be considered an endorsement from the trademark holder.

Introduction

Congratulations on downloading your copy of *Intermittent Fasting: Lose Fat, Build Muscle, and Get Fit.* Thank you for doing so.

Intermittent fasting has grown in popularity in recent years, thanks in large part to its ability to promote greater rates of nutrient absorption in the meals you eat.

It has also grown in popularity because it doesn't require adherents to change radically the types of foods you are eating, when you are eating, or even drastically alter the number of calories you consume in each 24-hour period.

In fact, the most common type of intermittent fasting is to simply consume two slightly larger than average meals during a day instead of the usual three.

This makes the intermittent fasting diet plan an ideal choice for those who find they have difficulty sticking to more stringent diet plans, as it only requires changing one habit, the number of meals per day, instead of many habits all at once.

Many people find that practicing intermittent fasting leads to real results.

It's simple enough to manage successfully over a prolonged period while at the same time being efficient enough to provide the type of results that can keep motivation levels high enough once the novelty of the new diet begins to fade.

The secret to intermittent fasting's success is the simple fact that your body behaves differently when it's in a fasting, versus a fed state.

When your body is in what is known as a fed state, it is actively digesting and absorbing food.

This begins some five minutes after you have finished putting food into your body, and can last anywhere from three to five hours depending on the how complicated the food is for your body to digest.

While in the fed state, your body is actively producing insulin which in turn makes it harder for it to burn fat properly.

The period after digestion has occurred, the insulin levels start dropping back towards normal which can take anywhere from 8 to 12 hours, and is the buffer between the fed and fasted state.

Once your insulin levels return to normal, the fasted state begins which is the period where your body can process fat most effectively.

Unfortunately, this means that many people never reach the point where they can burn fat most efficiently, as they rarely go eight hours, much less 12 hours from some type of caloric consumption.

There is hope! However, as to start seeing real results, all you need to do is break the three meal a day habit.

There are plenty of books on this subject on the market.

Thanks again for choosing this one.

Every effort was made to ensure it is full of as much useful information as possible.

Please enjoy!

Chapter 1: How Intermittent Fasting Works

History of Intermittent Fasting

Fasting is not a trend and has been a part of some religious beliefs including Buddhism, Islam, and Christianity.

Decades before this generation, the process may have been because of the unavailability of food resources.

Just remember, it is not a starvation diet since starvation is considered an involuntary absence of food.

Consider breakfast which is the most important time of your day. After all, it is 'break-fast'—which is a part of every day.

Fasting dates to the day of Hippocrates of Cos {c460 – c370BC} who is considered in many ideals as the father of modern medicine.

He stated, "To eat when you are sick is to feed your illness."

Plato, an ancient Greek thinker, and Aristotle, his student, were believers and supporters of fasting.

The Greeks believed that fasting is the "physician within."

This is the same logic/instinct portrayed by your pets.

Ben Franklin, an important founding father of America, also stated, "The best of all medicine is resting and fasting."

The Basics

Intermittent fasting is a way of eating to ensure that you get the most out of every meal you eat.

The core tenants of intermittent fasting mean that you don't need to change what you are eating.

Instead, you must change when you are eating it.

Intermittent fasting is a viable alternative to traditional diets or simply cutting your daily caloric intake which can help fasters lean up without changing the number of calories they consume in a day.

In fact, the preferred method of intermittent fasting is to simply eat two large meals every day instead of three (or more) meals in that same period.

Intermittent fasting is also a great option for those who traditionally have trouble sticking to diet plans since it only requires you to change one small habit, instead of several larger ones.

Intermittent fasting is extremely effective for most people because it is simple enough for them to attempt.

At the same time, it is efficient to warrant the task.

The key to understating why intermittent fasting is so successful lies in the differences in your body during a fasted state versus a fed state, as well as the important changes that will come across because of changing habits and sticking with it.

The body is considered to be in the fed state when it is in the process of absorbing and digesting food.

The fed state tends to start roughly five minutes after you begin eating, and lasting from three to five hours, depending on how long it takes your body to digest the meal.

A fed state, in turn, leads to higher levels of insulin which make it much more difficult for the body to burn fat.

The period directly after the fed sate is referred to as the post-absorptive state which is the period of time where the body is not actively processing food, and its insulin levels begin to fall.

This state lasts for between eight and twelve hours and directly precedes the fasted state.

The fasted state occurs between nine and twelve hours after the post-absorptive state and is the point where the body's insulin levels are at its lowest which in turn make it the period of time where the most fat can be burned during physical activity.

Unfortunately for many people, they rarely go twelve hours without eating which means that no matter how hard they exercise they are not burning fat as efficiently as possible.

However, this also means that you can burn fat and build muscle by simply altering your feeding habits.

Scientifically Proven

Your metabolic rate is increased with short-term fasting because of the hormonal changes ranging in categories of 3.6% to 14%.

Studies have established weight loss after three to twenty-four weeks on the intermittent fasting program to maintain losses of 3.0 to 8.0%.

In comparison to other studies on weight loss, these are high percentages that cannot be ignored.

In the same studies, many of the individuals lost 4.0 to 7.0% of his/her waist circumference.

This is an indication of how the harmful buildup of belly fat can cause disease and other issues around your organs.

You have to consider these results are from eating fewer overall calories, and not binging during the days off.

You must maintain a sensible eating program.

While the science behind intermittent fasting is certainly promising, there are a few things you will need to keep in mind when starting any new dietary plan.

No diet, regardless of how miraculous it appears, can help you if you don't obey a few golden rules:

- *Keep a calorie deficit:* While this is true for any diet, it is even more true for intermittent fasting since it can be so easy to overeat once you do eat in such a way that it negates any benefits you might have felt.

  Remember, you need to burn 3,500 calories weekly to lose one pound each week.

- *Maintain self-control:* Intermittent fasting only works if your body goes completely without food for at least twelve hours and any caloric intact resets the cycle.

  As such, it is extremely important to ensure that you maintain control of you bodily urges if you hope to see real results from this type of approach.

  Remember, fasting for at least twelve hours only allows you to eat normally or slightly more than an average meal, it does not give you license to eat everything in sight.

  Keeping your appetites in check is a strict requirement for success.

- *Be consistent:* Regardless of the type of weight loss that you ultimately choose to pursue, it is important to choose one and stick with it.

Attempting an intermittent fast for a few days before switching to another plan such as the Paleo diet before trying out a low-carb approach will only cause your body to freak out and hold on to every possible calorie until it figures out what in the world is happening.

Remember, fasting regularly and consistently is the surest way to see any of its benefits.

Only after your body has time to adjust to your new routine will it then be able to adapt appropriately.

It can begin to increase several positive enzymes and neural pathways to maximize weight loss using this method.

Consider consistency the ace-in-the-hole of proactive weight loss success.

Possible Side Effects:

While intermittent fasting has some scientifically proven benefits, it is not with its potential side effects.

The biggest one of these is the initial change in your bowel movements as periods of constipation or in some cases diarrhea could occur.

Fortunately, they should not last more than a few days as your body adjusts to the new method of caloric intake.

Additional damage can be done to the body if periods of fasting are routinely followed by periods of excessive binging.

It is important to attempt intermittent fasting, and your periods of eating after, in moderation.

If you notice any serious immediate physical changes after you begin any form of dieting regime, it is important to consult a nutritionist.

Chapter 2: Intermittent Types and Fasting Schedules

While the core ideas behind the various forms of intermittent fasting are all the same, there are quite a few different ways to go about it.

Your best bet is to try a few and see which one your body naturally responds to the easiest.

16:8 Method

This method involves fasting for 16 hours for men, or 14 hours for women, before allowing a reasonable number of calories for the remaining 8 to 10 hours.

During this period, you should only consume items that have zero calories including black coffee (a splash of cream is fine), water, diet soda, and sugar-free gum.

The easiest way to attempt this schedule is to stop eating after dinner in the evening and wait 14 or 16 hours from there.

This means skipping breakfast and picking things up in the early afternoon.

Again, the specifics of when you fast are not nearly as important as ensuring that you fast for the same period of time as regularly as possible.

If you vary your fasting period too much, it can lead to an erratic change in your hormones, which among other things; make it much more difficult for your body to shed any excess weight.

If you find yourself without the time required to eat a proper meal to break the fast normally, ensure you at least eat something to keep your body on the correct cycle.

If you are exercising, as well as intermittently fasting, it is important to ensure that you are eating more carbohydrates than fats while you are working out, while on days you are not exercising the opposite is true.

It is important to ensure that every day you keep your protein intake at a steady level.

Stay away from processed foods whenever possible.

One of the biggest benefits of this type of fasting is that it's extremely flexible so that it will work for a wide variety schedules.

Most people find it helpful to either eat two large meals during the 8 or 10-hour period feeding period or split that time into three smaller meals as that is the way most people are already programmed.

On days you are exercising as well as fasting, it is important to try and always break your fast with a mix of protein, vegetables, and fruit.

If you generally go to the gym directly after you have broken your fast, it is important to include enough carbohydrates to give your muscles the energy they need to get the most out of your workout.

If you are planning to exercise, it is usually best to start the early afternoon healthy with a medium calorie meal.

Then, exercise within three hours before eating a larger meal soon afterward.

In this larger meal, it is important to add a larger portion of complex carbohydrates.

You can even have a little dessert as long as it is in moderation. Remember, fasting is different than dieting.

On days you do not plan on exercising, it is important to adjust your caloric intake appropriately.

Start by limiting your carbohydrate intake, and instead focus on eating lots of protein, dark green, leafy vegetables and fruit in moderation.

Unlike on days you are exercising, the first meal you eat on rest days should be your largest regarding caloric intake with this one meal counting for about 40 percent of your daily total.

Remember, during this meal, you should be taking in more protein than anything else.

For your final meal during rest days, it is important to include a protein source that will take lots of time to digest which in turn means it will keep you full for more of your fast the following morning.

It also provides the body with enough stored amino acids to prevent it from breaking down muscle during the fast.

Eat-Stop-Eat

This form of fasting can be considered the most beneficial to those who are already eating healthy but want to give their weight loss an extra boost.

On this type of program, you don't eat anything one or two days a week.

During this period, you should only consume things that have zero calories including black coffee (a splash of cream is fine), water, diet soda, and sugar-free gum.

When you are finished fasting, it is important not to eat too much more than normal and always to avoid binging as extended periods of fast/binge cycles can cause serious damage to your body.

As always, it is important to practice moderation and self-control to get the most out of the fasting cycle.

This fast cycle works on the assumption that in to lose a pound of weight a week, all you need to do is give up 3,500 calories.

So, it might be best to get it out of the way in two quick bursts rather than fasting for a portion of every single day.

This fasting plan emphasizes resistance weight training for maximum benefits.

Going a full day without eating can be difficult for some people at first, but it is perfectly acceptable to work up to a full day of fasting by holding out as long as possible and increasing that amount of time with practice.

A good way to start is by choosing days that you know don't have any prior food commitments.

Beginning a fasting program on a day when you know you have a lunch meeting is just a bad idea.

When first starting this fast cycle, fatigue, headaches or feelings of anger or anxiousness are all common side-effects and should be considered a good stopping point for your current fast.

These side-effects will diminish as your body adjusts to the new cycle.

After going a full day without any calories, it will be natural to have the desire to binge during your fist meal.

You must have the self-control to fight these urges since not only is binging bad for you; it can easily undo all your hard work from the previous 24 hours. Practice self-discipline and make your fasting worth the effort.

The Warrior Diet

The Warrior Diet takes the 16:8 Program and kicks it up a notch by recommending that you fast for roughly 20 hours out of each day followed by one meal where you get all your calories in the four remaining hours of the day.

This form of intermittent fasting follows the belief that humans are naturally nocturnal eaters.

Therefore, eating at night helps the body more easily process the nutrients it needs.

In this case, fasting is a bit of a misnomer as during the 20-hour period you are allowed to eat a serving of raw vegetables or fruits and maybe a serving of protein if you just can't otherwise continue.

This works because it causes the body's natural sympathetic nervous system to activate a flight or fight response which in turns increases your natural levels of alertness, and increases energy while at the same time increasing the amount of fat burned.

The large meal each evening then allows the body to focus on repairing itself and improving its muscles.

When following the Warrior Diet, it is important to start each evening meal with vegetables, followed by protein, fat, and carbohydrates.

This form of fasting is popular for two reasons.

First, the fact that a few small and reasonable snacks are allowed during the fasting process making this type of fasting attractive to those who are attempting the practice for the first time.

Second, nearly everyone who attempts this form of fasting reports a significant amount of increased energy throughout the day as well as increase in the amount of fat lost per week.

On the other hand, the relatively strict nature of this diet can make it difficult for some people to follow for long periods of time.

The timing of the large meal can also make it difficult for some people to follow because it can naturally interfere with some social engagements.

Finally, some people don't like having to eat their food in a specific order.

Try it for yourself and see what works for you.

Fat Loss Forever

This form of intermittent fasting combines elements of several other styles of fasting to create something rather unique.

The good news is that you get a cheat day every week.

The bad news is that it is followed by a one and a half day fast with the remainder of the week being split between 16:8 and 20:4 fasting.

For this diet, it is important to schedule your exercise rest days for the second part of the 36-hour cycle.

Otherwise, it is important to stay as busy on these days as possible to help combat your hunger.

If you find it hard to control your appetite on cheat days, then this form of intermittent fasting may not be for you since it requires you to go from sixty to zero quickly and regularly.

Also, it is important not to try and last 36 hours without eating food all at once.

You will need to build up your body's tolerance for fasting.

As such, it is usually better to start with another form of intermittent fasting and work up to the Fat Loss Forever method after your body has already gotten out of the habit of eating every three or four hours.

Remember to always fast responsibly, and never push your body to the point where you feel physically ill.

Also, remember it is important to fast on a routine to allow your body the time it needs to adjust to the change.

Alternate Day Diet

This form of intermittent fasting actually means you never have to go long without food, if you so choose.

Every other day you eat normally, and on the off-days, you simply consume one-fifth of the calories you consume on the normal days.

The average daily caloric consumption is between 2,000 and 2,500 calories which mean that the average off-day varies between 400 and 500 calories.

If you enjoy exercising every day, then this form of intermittent fasting may not be for you since you will have to severely limit your workouts on off-days.

When you first start this form of intermittent fasting, the easiest way to make it through the low-calorie days is by trying any one of a variety of protein shakes.

It is important to work back to 'real' natural foods on these days because they will always be healthier than the shakes.

This form of intermittent fasting is all about losing weight.

Those who try it tend to average between two and three pounds lost per week.

If you attempt the Alternate Day Diet, it is extremely important to eat regularly on your full-calorie days.

Binging will not only negate any progress you have made, but it can also cause serious damage to your body if continued over time.

Irregularly Skipping Meals

If you are interested in trying out the benefits of intermittent fasting for yourself, but you have an irregular schedule or are not sure if it is for you, then skipping a meal or two now and then may be the type of intermittent fasting for you.

As previously discussed, getting into a fasting routine is important to see the maximum results for your effort, but that doesn't mean occasionally fasting doesn't come with some benefits as well.

What's more, once you have tried skipping a meal now and then you can see for yourself just how easy it is which in turn can lead to more positive changes down the line.

With so many intermittent fasting options available the odds are good that one fits your schedule, so give it a try. What have you got to lose (besides a few pounds)?

Chapter 3: Health Benefits

Other than weight loss, you can receive benefits from intermittent fasting in many other ways.

You will live a longer life from achieving an extended fasting state and diverting your energy while improving your biological functions.

Just remember, the plan will not in any way cause you to starve.

The emergency signals transported by your body is simply that—a signal.

The fasting state your body is experiencing will diminish once your body adjusts to the diet method of intermittent fasting you choose to take.

These are some of the crucial elements to consider:

- *Brain Health:* Your brain hormone—BDNF—also known as brain-derived "neurotropic" factor—is a protein that can aid in the growth of new nerve cells.

  It is also believed to provide protection against Alzheimer's and Parkinson's disease.

- *Cancer:* Studies using animals have suggested intermittent fasting can be beneficial in the prevention of cancer.

- *Heart Health:* The blood triglycerides, LDL cholesterol, insulin resistance, and blood sugar can be reduced using this plan.

Each of these presents a huge risk element for heart ailments or disease.

- *Inflammation:* Chronic diseases are driven by inflammation, and the fasting plans help to reduce the inflammation as proven by private studies.

  Your body will be capable of repairing, healing, and recovering more quickly than without the diet plan.

- *Insulin Resistance:* Your blood sugar levels can be lowered by 3.0% to 3.6 as fasting insulin levels can also decrease as much as 20% to 31%.

  These figures indicate you should be better sheltered against type 2 diabetes as well as a more continuous level of mood and energy stages.

- *Anti-Aging:* The process has only been tested using animals, but the rats tested lived 36% to 83% longer than ones that were not fasting.

- *Lower Stress Levels:* The cortisol production is lowered.

- *Fatty Acid Oxidation:* Your body will burn more fats as energy with the oxidation process and will also provide quick weight loss.

Note: Each of these studies are in early stages.

More research needs to be provided using human testing during the fasting process.

Chapter 4: The Process

While intermittent fasting is undeniably beneficial, it can be difficult to get started or to see through to the point where your body adapts to a new schedule.

The following tips and tricks can help set you on the path to success.

Have a conversation with yourself:

Intermittent fasting has a wide variety of proven benefits, but it is not for everyone.

Before you attempt a fast, it is important to have a real dialogue with yourself.

Consider your level of self-discipline, your current attachment to food, any regular activities that would make fasting difficult or awkward, your general lifestyle, and your level of exercise.

Deciding to try a different fitness regime is a lot easier on day one, than after struggling through a week or more of faulty fasting.

Watch your response:

While it is important to keep tabs on how your body is responding to intermittent fasting, it is doubly important to monitor your vitals during the initial phase when your body is adjusting to the new feeding times.

Some discomfort is to be expected for the first three to four weeks, but anything longer or more severe should be discussed with a doctor as soon as possible.

The early days will have ups and downs:

While your body adjusts to intermittent fasting, there will be times where you are losing weight and times where your body is trying to hold on to every calorie it has.

This is natural and to be expected as your body realigns its hormone levels.

Drink lots of water:

Not only will water help you feel full throughout your fast, staying hydrated is akin to staying healthy.

Aim for at least a gallon of water per day.

Caffeine naturally suppresses the appetite:

Black coffee works best as there is little to it which can negatively affect your metabolism or general wellbeing.

The same cannot be said for most 0-calorie caffeinated beverages.

Artificial sweeteners have been shown to cause some health problems.

Still, anything with caffeine will help calm your appetite for at least a little while.

Keep yourself busy:

Ensure that the latter parts of your fast aren't just spent waiting around to eat.

Intermittent fasting has the possibility to be either extremely difficult or surprisingly easy depending solely on how much of the time you spend thinking about food.

Find ways to occupy your mind, and you will be surprised how quickly meal time will roll around.

Start each fast off right:

At the start of your fast, your body will still have the most fuel in its system to work with, which is why it is best to start each fast with the most difficult items on your to-do list.

As you move farther and farther from the last period of time, and you take in fresh calories, your thought processes will naturally begin to slow in your body's effort to save energy.

Difficult tasks will inherently seem easier when your body is working at maximum efficiency.

Make it work for you:

Intermittent fasting can work around any type of schedule which is part of what makes it so great.

If you find yourself feeling trapped by the period of time you are allowing yourself to eat, why don't you move it?

Fasting should be about adding freedom to your schedule, not restraining it.

Don't expect results overnight:

As previously discussed, it will take some time for your body to adjust fully to your new dietary patterns, and for it to start reflecting these new results.
Try intermittent fasting regularly for at least a month before rendering judgment on the success of the plan.

Vary your schedule:

After you have given your body time to adjust to an intermittent fasting schedule, it is important to take the time to fluctuate your on/off patterns throughout the day to see what works best for you.

Taking the time to experiment may yield unexpected results.

Start slow:

If you find that you are having difficulty starting the transition to an intermittent fasting program full bore, try moving your breakfast time back one hour each week.

Before you know it, you will have reached a 16:8 or 14:10 split without even trying.

Keep it to yourself:

While there is plenty of scientific evidence that supports intermittent fasting, there are still plenty of skeptics out there.

That negativity isn't something you need, especially when you are first starting out.

After you have started seeing results for yourself, it will be much easier to defend the process to non-believers.

Just show them a before and after picture.

Start the day off with a belly full of liquid:

Often the signals for hunger and the signals for thirst can get crossed in your brain.

After it has sent out enough ignored thirst signals, it starts sending out hunger signals instead.

As such, starting the morning off by drinking at least half a liter of water is an excellent way to quench your body's thirst from the past seven or eight hours.

It should be enough to keep you feeling full for at least a few extra hours each morning.

Don't take on too much, too fast:

Even if you think you feel fine when you first begin an intermittent fast cycle, it is important to always give your body the time it needs to recover.

Never go more than two days out of a week without eating.

There is an important distinction between fasting and starving yourself.

Splurge when you want:

Remember that you need to burn 3,500 calories to lose a pound a week, but how you do that is up to you.

If you want to have a particularly appetizing dessert or unhealthy main course, that is perfectly fine, as long as you make an effort to make up the difference throughout the week.

Distract yourself:

Distraction is especially important as your body is adapting to your new eating habits, and becomes increasingly important the farther into a fast you go.

Try going out and being active when you are struggling with the plan to help refocus your thinking patterns.

Besides, the exercise also helps push away the pounds.

Add protein to your meals:

There is nothing better at combating hunger than protein, plain and simple.

It is also great for building lean muscle.

If you find yourself unable to get through even 10 hours without eating, then it might be a sign that you should add more protein to your diet.

Try Branched Chain Amino Acids:

For those on a low-calorie diet such as intermittent fasting, studies show that a BCAA supplement will stimulate additional fat loss while at the same time preventing lean muscle from being consumed as the body tries to feed itself.

Intermittent fasting is not an excuse to eat poorly:

Intermittent fasting works on the principle that eating fewer calories than you burn is a surefire way to lose weight.
This theory falls apart if you use the fact that you are fasting as an excuse to eat nothing but junk food when you are eating.

Self-control and self-discipline are both equally important when it comes to eating properly. Intermittent fasting has a wide variety of health benefits.

Why not accentuate them even more with a healthy diet to go along with it?

Break your fast the right way:

The content and quality of your first meal of the day can easily set the tone for those that follow.

Use this to your advantage, and start your feeding window off right with something fit and healthy.

You will be surprised at how much this improves your willpower for later meals.

Consider the difference between head hunger and body hunger:

As you get used to the process of intermittent fasting, you will become acquainted with several different types of hunger and ultimately learn how to tell when you are truly hungry as opposed to just habitually used to eating.

While it will initially be difficult to tell the difference, you will come to know them both intimately in time.

Learn what your body is saying:

While many people consider a sudden craving for a particular type of food as an indication that they are hungry, and take action to respond accordingly.

This, in fact, is often just a craving brought on by an ancient part of the brain which equates things that are salty, sweet, and high in fat as vital parts of a regular diet.

Since once upon a time, having those three qualities equated to things that were high in positive nutrients as well.

This is no longer the case and tends to be the opposite these days.

As such, these types of urges can safely be ignored.

Take the time to investigate a sudden surge of hunger to see if it could instead be related to your emotional state instead of your physical one.

Exercise in moderation:

Dieting works by ensuring that you are taking in fewer calories than you are burning in a fixed period of time.

As such, if you are trying one of the intermittent fasting options that involve you not eating for a day or more, then it is extremely important to ensure that you adjust your exercise plan for these days as well.

When exercising, your body requires fuel. It will take it from your muscles if you don't give it another choice.

Exercising too much while you're fasting is a guaranteed recipe for disaster.

Don't cover real issues with fasting:

Those with a penchant for eating disorders or those who believe they might be should stay away for intermittent fasting as it can easily lead to more serious issues if not controlled properly.

Remember, it is important to have the willpower to stop eating for a set period of time, but it is also equally important to have the willpower to begin eating again once the fast is over.

Chapter 5: Weight Loss and Intermittent Fasting

You need to understand what your daily calorie needs will be to adopt a realistic diet plan and maintain a new desirable weight.

The use of an adult <u>BMI and Calorie Calculator</u> will be an essential tool if the calories are not indicated in the recipe.

Most products you purchase will have ingredient panels listing the counts, so you will have a general idea of how to plan your menu around your intermittent fasting plan.

You will need to enter your sex, height, weight, and age into the calculator.

You will also need to provide the calculator with your daily activity schedule (such as daily—more than an hour—less than an hour—or rarely.

The BMI will indicate your BMI score and the amount of calories necessary to maintain your current body weight.

It will make your goals simpler to map by providing you with the tallies from your calculations to lower your counts.

Maintain a Healthy Diet Plan

The components for a healthier eating pattern using intermittent fasting methods will account for all the beverages and foods within a suitable calorie level.

A good plan for a healthy fasting pattern will include the following:

- Whole Fruits

- Oils

- Grains (a minimum of half should be whole grains)

- Protein foods such as eggs, poultry, lean meats, seafood, nuts, seeds, and soy products

- Varied veggies from all the main subgroups include—starchy legumes (peas and beans), red and orange, dark green and others.

Health concerns in the United States are focused on fundamental elements that should be limited when using the intermittent fasting diet plan.

They recommend you do the following:

- Consume less than 10% of your daily calories from saturated fats.

- Eat less than 10% of your daily intake of calories from added sugars.

- Sodium consumption should be less than 2,300 mg (milligrams).

- Moderation must be accompanied if you consume alcohol products.

  You should have no more than one daily if you are a woman and only two each day if you are a man.

What Not to Eat

With all the talk of the importance of natural foods, what foods should I avoid to make my intermittent fast more effective?

As a general rule, the following foods should be avoided or at least limited as much as possible.

- *Processed Meats:* While protein is an undeniably important part of a healthy diet, seeking your protein from meats which have been processed will stuff your body so full of chemicals that any benefits the meal might have had are otherwise lost.

  These meats tend to be lower in protein while higher in sodium and preservatives that can cause a variety of health risks, including asthma and heart disease, than the quality of the cuts of meat found in most grocery stores.

- *Non-organic potatoes:* While starch and the carbohydrates they contain are an important part of a balanced meal, non-organic potatoes are not worth the trouble.

  They are treated with chemicals while still in the ground.

  They are treated again before they head to the store to ensure they stay "fresh" as long as possible.

  These chemicals have been shown to increase the risk of health issues like autism, asthma, birth defects, learning disabilities, Parkinson's and Alzheimer's disease as well as multiple types of cancer.

- *Farm-raised salmon:* Much like processed meat, farm-raised salmon are the least healthy type of an otherwise healthy meal choice.

  When salmon are raised in tubs near one another for a prolonged period of time, they lose much of their natural vitamin D while picking up traces of PCB, DDT, carcinogens, and bromine.

  Choose wild caught fish if possible.

- *Non-organic milk:* Despite being touted as part of a balanced diet, non-organic milk is routinely found to be full of growth hormones as well as puss as a result of over-milking the cows.

  The growth hormones leave behind antibiotics which can, in turn, make it more difficult for the human body to counter infections as well as causing an increased chance of colon cancer, prostate cancer, and breast cancer.

- *White Flour:* Much like processed meats, by the time white flour is done being produced; it is completely devoid of any nutritional value.

  When eaten as part of a regular diet, white flour has been shown to increase a woman's chance of breast cancer by a shocking 200 percent.

These are just a few of the reasons that processed foods should be considered a problem in the modern world.

Processed foods can be considered any items which contain preservatives, chemical colors, flavorings, additives or chemicals which change its texture.

An additional extremely important warning sign of unhealthy food is when an item contains a large amount of carbohydrates in their refined form.

The cliff-notes version is this, the sooner you begin to take the time to read labels and check ingredients, the sooner you can start getting the most out of the meals you eat in between intermittent fasting sessions. Making a real, consciousness effort to do so may very well be the difference between life and death.

Chapter 6: Intermittent Fasting and Nutrition

How to Boost Your Metabolism

With all the hard work for your intermittent fasting, it is always good to know there are other ways to speed up the process at the same time.

It is good to know these are some of the specific foods you should eat to help the metabolism process of losing weight:

Protein-Rich Food Groups

Your body will need more energy to digest these products:

- Eggs
- Seeds and nuts
- Legumes
- Fish
- Meat
- Fish

The thermic effect of food is referred to as TEF which is the number of calories required by your body to absorb/digest the nutrients received by your meals.

The protein intake will also make you have a full feeling much longer, and possibly prevent you from overeating.

Essential Vitamins and Minerals

Zinc, iron, and selenium are essential for your healthy body functions.

It is shown by research a diet low in these elements reduces the ability of the thyroid gland to produce crucial hormones.

This process will significantly slow the metabolism down.

It is best to eat seeds, nuts, legumes, meat, and seafood.

- *Chili Peppers:* The chemical found in chili peppers is called capsaicin which will boost your metabolism.

  The capsaicin will increase the fat and calories you burn during your intermittent fasting plan.

  Twenty research studies indicated you would lose/burn approximately fifty extra calories daily.

  However, now all researchers agree with the theory.

  At any rate, enjoy the chili peppers.

- *Pulses and Legumes:* This food group includes peanuts, lentils, chickpeas, beans, and peas which are extremely high in protein levels in comparison to other plant foods.

  According to research studies, your higher protein counts will require your body to burn a larger number of calories to digest them, versus the lower-protein foods.

  Recent studies have indicated participants who consumed a legume-rich diet for eight weeks increased the metabolism rate and lost more than 1.5 times more weight versus the other controlled group of applicants.

- *Coffee:* Your caffeine levels can help increase the metabolic rate by approximately 11%.

Studies have shown consumption of a minimum of 270 mg of caffeine—about three cups of coffee—will burn away an additional 100 calories daily.

The rates can surely boost your intermittent fasting as long as you leave it sugar-free.

- *Tea:* Tea is offered as a good source of beverage because of the catechins in the tea conglomerate with the caffeine to help speed up your metabolism.

  The catechins are an antioxidant and a type of natural phenol which is from the chemical family of flavonoids.

  An additional 100 calories can be burned daily to increase your metabolism by four to ten percent with the use of green and oolong tea.

  The effects may be different with each fasting participant.

Chapter 7: Different Methods for Everyday Living

Method 16:8 or the Lean Gains Diet Plan

Another term for this plan is the Lean Gains protocol which implicates for a time slot of eight hours that you can eat a restricted diet and fast for the remainder time of sixteen hours for men and fourteen hours for women.

Hugh Jackman was the emblem used to discover the facts and make the headlines.

The 16:8 method for intermittent fasting is the most preferred method for weight loss—besides you will be sleeping for approximately eight of those fasting hours.

On the remainder eight to ten hours, the meals should be slightly larger while still relatively health conscious.

The fasting period allows for zero calorie consumption.

If you are overweight and have a sedentary lifestyle; you should avoid most of the starchy carbohydrates.

You have to cram all of your calories in that time allotment to ensure the successes of the plan.

Many individuals on the plan can fit two filling meals into the eight to ten-hour time frame or three regular meals if desired.

Once again, the most important element is consistency.

A study was performed by the Obesity Society stating if you have your dinner before 2:00 p.m., your hunger yearnings will be reduced for the remainder of the day.

At the same time, your fat-burning reserves are boosted.

No matter what you have heard about this plan, you will not be as hungry once you have the plan and your menu scheduled.

That is the secret to a slimmer body, get the counts right.

Another advantage is that you can begin the plate at any time that suits your schedule.

You can use these sample menus as a basis for your plan:

Day 1

- **Morning:** Tea, water, or coffee is allowed with a small amount of milk or heavy cream

- **Lunch:** Chicken Breast/black bean sauce, green veggies, and fruit.

- **Dinner:** Salmon and baked veggies with one potato. (If this is too much for one meal, break it in half and eat it later.

Day 2: Repeat Day 1

Additional Tips

- *Sugar Substitutes:* Xylitol can replace sugar. Replace the coffee with black or green tea (advisable if you like the tastes).

- *Stay Hydrated:* Drink plenty of tea, water, or coffee during the morning hours. It also helps prevent the pangs of hunger you will feel. If possible, replace the coffee with black or green tea.

- *Sleep:* You need to have a full eight hours of sleep. It is advisable to avoid your cell phone and laptop (blue light) for up to an hour before you are ready to retire for the evening.

The Consistent Path

The goal is to set your eating schedule to the same time daily to program our body.

If you vary during the fasting plan, your hormones will be all over the place, resulting in your body holding onto the weight instead of detaching from the extra pounds.

It is also important to keep your protein on an even kilter throughout your fasting schedule.

For women, it should remain at 55 grams daily.

For men, it should be in the area of 60 grams daily.

If you consume the correct levels of protein and exercise regularly while taking in a steady amount of carbs, you should have all the energy needed on a daily basis.

However, if you are less inclined to exercise you should focus on healthy fats while you minimize the carbs.

Aim for approximately 0.7 grams of healthy fats for each pound of body weight daily.

As with the other plans, it is best to avoid processed foods and unhealthy fats while searching for healthier—natural alternatives when possible.

If you are not an avid exerciser, you also need to adjust your meals for the days to ensure you don't overeat accidentally.

Eat-Stop-Eat

Once or twice each week, you will fast for twenty-four hours.

As an illustration, you would eat dinner one morning and not eat again until the following morning.

Most professionals say if you make it to twenty hours; it's okay.

To further condition your body, for two days eat about 2,500 calories if you are a man and 2,000 if you are a woman.

After several regular eating days, attempt another fasting, and repeat the agenda.

Non-Fasting and Fasting Day Nutrients

For the days on an active fast, try not to consume many calories.

You can drink sparkling or plain water, diet soda, coffee, or tea.

When the fast is complete, eat what you like using restraint.

Enjoy plenty of veggies, fruits, and take advantage of the spices for variety.

Protein should be apparent using twenty to thirty grams of high-quality protein.

Consume a total of one-hundred grams every four to five hours.

You can use protein powders if needed.

If you are gaining extra pounds in between your fasting schedule, consider cutting back by approximately 10% on the amount of food you consume on non-fasting days.

Some individuals cannot 'hack' the plan and state it makes him/her less adaptable to enjoying time with friends at social gatherings.

Many have issues of crankiness and headaches which can lead to the plan's failure.

With that said, the plan's benefits are overwhelming because you can judge your progress, and you choose to eat.

It takes learning some self-control, but you can get it.

Note: Never fast two consecutive days. Also, you should not take the challenge more than two fasting days in one week.

Fluid Intake

With a strict plan such as this one, you must remain hydrated.

You can drink plenty of clear liquids, but where are the nutrients?

On your fasting days, stick to apple juice, water, broth, cranberry juice, ice pops, plain gelatin, black coffee or tea.

This is okay since you will be fasting for twenty to twenty-four hours.

You can also enjoy foods including ice cream, skim milk, juice with pulp, or strained creamy soup.

Try a whey protein supplemental shake or some low-fat frozen yogurt.

These choices will provide some essential nutrients, fiber, as well as the necessary calorie counts.

Just be sure to use low-calorie juices, ice cream, and a few ice cubes for a smoothie treat.

It is advisable to confer with your physician before you begin this or any other dieting plan.

While you are fasting, you might need to discontinue any dietary supplements or medications.

According to research at Vanderbilt University, daily liquid diets will provide you between 400 to 800 calories.

Additional Tips

With this fasting method, it is essential to not fall into a habit of fasting and binging because it will create havoc within your body.

It is more than your body can handle since the cycle will only work for individuals who can practice control and moderate consumption of food.

It is recommended by the professionals to perform resistance-style weight training on the days you aren't fasting.

Try a minimal yoga session or light cardio exercise if you feel completely out of it on your fasting days.

Any more vigorous exercising could make it difficult to achieve the time allotment of your fasting schedule.

Remember, at first—it is common to feel angered, anxious, fatigued, or have headaches.

This will pass once your body adjusts to the new dieting plan.

Try to keep in mind that every single day you can successfully stay on your desired plan is one more day toward your successful goal.

The Warrior Diet

It is believed that the name of the diet is a reflection of the ancient ancestors who were natural nocturnal eaters.

As a step up from the Lean Gains diet and as a variation of the daily fast; the Warrior Diet is a plan promoting one healthy meal daily—usually dinner.

The method is parallel with the human 24-hour rhythm and can encourage excellent general health while removing the harmful toxins from your body.

You should try to eat at least several hours before going to sleep for the night.

The Daytime Feeding Schedule

For the plan to be effective, you need to consume less food during the daytime hours.

Eat small servings of veggies, fruits, and a protein such as a yogurt, whey protein, or kefir.

Sidestep consumption of meats, grains, refined foods (pasta, corn tortillas, etc.) which lack the nutrient and are usually processed foods. Also, avoid sugary beverages and treats.

Every few hours, you should eat a small serving of protein or fruit.

Eat green veggies such as celery, leafy greens, cucumbers, and peppers which are not restricted to your intake amounts.

Nighttime Feeding Frenzy

You can eat as much food as you wish but keep the correct food combinations. Enlist as many different aromas, colors, and textures to create new taste sensations for your evening meal.

Eliminate or avoid using white vinegar.

When you feel full or have satisfied your hunger or if you become more thirsty than hungry; it is time to stop eating.

Follow the Rules

Start off with your salad, protein, and veggies and complete the meal with a few fats or carbs.

Take a short twenty-minute break after the protein and vegetables which will be a signal to your brain to recharge your appetite.

If you are still hungry, continue your meal.

Organic foods are the best choices which will include grass-fed, free range, and hormone free animal products.

Your eggs, dairy, and meat, as well as your fish consumption, should be a 'wild' catch.

Processed sugars are considered toxic on this diet plan.

You should also exercise as a critical step in your fasting plan.

After your workout, consume 20 to 30 grams of net protein with no additional sugar.

Guidelines for Success

Remember to plan your menus ahead of time to be sure you have the right combination of foods.

Vegetables and protein will combine with your entire menu planning needs. Starch, sugar, and fat cannot conglomerate effectively.

Examples of the Right Combinations

- Eggs and beans

- Seeds and nuts

- Eggs and potatoes

- Berries and Whey protein

- Cocoa nibs and peanut butter

- Potatoes and peas

- Nuts and wine

- Cheese and wine

- Rice and beans

Examples of the Wrong Combinations

- Pasta and wine

- Pasta and nuts

- Raisins and nuts (trail mix)

- Sugar and cream

- Jelly and peanut butter

- Jam and bread

- Granola (honey nut)

- Sour cream and potatoes

Sample Plan: Daytime Options

Early Morning: Tea, coffee, or cacao (no sugar) whole milk

Mid-morning: Vegetable juice or one fruit (8 ounces of berries)

Lunchtime: Salad with tomatoes, peppers, mixed greens, mushroom, onions, sprouts, and cucumber

Dressing for the salad: Use a small amount of olive oil OR whey protein

Afternoon: Fresh Fruit or Vegetable juice

Sample Plan: Nighttime Meal

For your one large meal of the day try some of the following food groups:

Protein: Eggs (cooked or poached), wild catch fish, organic cheeses such as goat and cottage

Cooked Veggies: Grilled or steamed cauliflower, broccoli, zucchini, onion, spinach, okra, and mushroom

Raw Veggies: Broccoli sprouts, salad greens, as well as red, yellow, and orange vegetables

Carbs: Use puree from butternut squash, carrots, Brussels sprouts, turnips, pumpkin, or cauliflower (steamed rooted veggies)

Use modest amounts of aged cheese, olive paste, parmesan cheese, or goat feta to top off your protein and vegetables.

During the detox meals, you can also reduce stress with green tea and berberine.

The berberine is a supplement to help unlock your metabolism to help balance your blood sugar levels during the detox diet plan.

The warrior diet is one of the most popular plans because it allows a sensible number of snacks to the daily routine which makes it more appealing to beginners on the fasting path.

The amount of energy will naturally get your body in the habit of burning fat for fuel.

Every-Other-Day Diet Plan

The alternate days using this plan was established by an assistant professor, Dr. Krista Varady, from the University of Illinois.

Women should consume between 500 to 600 calories, and men need to consume more than 400 to 500 calories daily.

However, on the feast day, you can eat anything you want and as much as you want.

The plan takes some planning since the diet begins between the hours of noon and 2 pm. These are some of the items to make your day more enjoyable:

The following meal will supply you with roughly 475 calories—depending on the type of soup used.

- ½ cup cooked chicken cooked without the skin and topped/Lemon juice/Fresh-ground pepper

- Bowl of tomato or low-sodium vegetable soup

- 1 ¼ cups of fruit salad

For Men Only: You can have a whole-wheat roll (medium 96-calorie) for a total of 566 calories.

Prepare the salad with pears strawberries, mandarin orange segments, and melon.

Enjoy Lean Beef
Choose a lean piece of beef cut similar to sirloin or tenderloin steak, and enjoy some low-calorie side dishes.

The basics of the plan are calculated for women.

For men, add 80 additional calories with a one-cup serving of asparagus with a teaspoon of olive oil for the topping.

For the remainder of the meal, enjoy a three-ounce seared steak with some onions.

Top it off with a bit of blue cheese.

Serve it with one cup of chard sautéed in 1 teaspoon of olive oil along with a ½ cup of polenta (cornmeal).

Use some lemon juice for seasoning.

Substitute with Seafood:
You need to consume some omega-3 fatty acids to remain heart-healthy.

For men, boost the counts to 553 by enjoying one cup of kale that has been sautéed with olive oil for an additional 102 calories.

Flavor the kale with crushed red pepper, red wine vinegar, and garlic.

For a woman (451 calories) enjoy three ounces of sautéed shrimp with jalapenos, garlic, onions, and some tomatoes (fresh and diced) on a bed of ½ cup of brown rice.

Place it all in a six-inch corn tortilla.

Also, have ¼ of an avocado (chopped) for dessert.

The Choice of No Meat:
Women can choose a meatless meal with 473 calories using a whole-wheat pizza crust.

As toppings use some black beans, diced tomatoes, barbecue sauce, fresh corn, and shredded mozzarella cheese.

Have a bowl of butternut squash soup, made using ¾ cup of fruit sorbet and veggie stock.

Men can veg-out with one cup of cauliflower salad for an extra 48 calories using reduced-fat mayonnaise.

He could also add ½ cup fruit such as blueberries, ½ cup yogurt if desired.

It is best to use the lower fat plain yogurt with the meal.

A Week's Worth of Planning

The logic behind this weekly regimen example involves eating 300 calories on the low-calorie days but can increase to 400 calories if you have an exercise plan in motion.

On the brighter side; women can eat 1200 to 1800 calories on the usual days.

The Low-Calorie Count Days

Day One:

Breakfast

- 1 small slice of deli meat

- 1 six-ounce glass of tomato juice

- ½ cup strawberries

Morning Snack Time
- ¼ cup mixed berries

- 1 tablespoon whey protein

- Blend the ingredients with 3 ice cubes and a cup of water

Lunch
- 1-ounce low-fat cheese

- ½ cup of pickles

- 1-six-ounce cup of tomato juice

Afternoon Snack Time
- 1 tablespoon salad dressing (calorie-free) on one celery stalk

-

Dinner Time
- Make an omelet using three egg whites, mushrooms, green peppers, and onions.

- For dessert have ½ cup of strawberries

Evening Snack
- Whey protein smoothie is your savior to enjoy with a cup of mixed veggies.

Normal Calorie Counted Days

Day 2:

Breakfast
- 1 small banana

- 20 Blueberries

- 1 English muffin (whole wheat) with 2 ¼ teaspoons of peanut butter

- 2/3 cup fat-free yogurt

Morning Snack Time
- 3 saltines

- 1 reduced-fat string cheese stick

Lunch
- 3 tablespoons of hummus with tomato and lettuce

- 1 Whole wheat wrap

- *Dessert*: 1 cup low-fat yogurt and ½ cup of applesauce

Afternoon Snack Time
- 15 almonds

Dinner
- 3 ounces—chicken breast

- 1 cup of broccoli and 2/3 cup of couscous

Evening Snacks
- 1 tablespoon peanut butter on 2 large graham cracker squares

Low-Calorie Day

Day 3:

Breakfast Meal
- ½ fruit serving

- 1-ounce of protein

- 1 six-ounce glass of tomato juice

Mid-morning Snack
- ¼ of a serving of fruit

- *Smoothie:* Combine three pieces of ice + one cup of water with one tablespoon whey protein.

Lunch Menu
- 1-ounce of protein

- 1 six-ounce glass of tomato juice

Mid-afternoon Snack
- Enjoy something under 50 calories.

Dinner Meal
- No more than 100 calories—include protein, veggies, and fruit as a focus point

Normal Calorie Count Day

Day 4:

Breakfast Meal
- 20 blueberries

- ¼ cup banana

- Whole wheat English muffin with 1 tablespoon of peanut butter

Mid-morning Snack
- 2 tablespoons of light cheese

- 3 rye crackers

Lunch
- 6 whole wheat crackers

- 1 cup of vegetable beef soup

- 1 piece fresh fruit

Mid-Afternoon Snack
- 5-6 medium strawberries

- 1-ounce dark chocolate

Dinner Menu
Steak and Peppers

Grill or broil:
1—four-ounce flank steak flavored with pepper and salt

Sauté Pepper Mixture:

- 2 teaspoons red wine

- 1 teaspoon olive oil

- ¼ cup onion sliced

- ¾ cup sliced bell pepper

- 1 tablespoon hoisin sauce

Instructions

1. Over a medium heat setting, sauté each of the ingredients listed using the teaspoon of olive oil.

2. After the flank steak is cooked to your preference, add the sautéed pepper mixture.

Calories: 267 per serving

Method 5:2 and 4:3

For this plan, you would eat a regular diet for five days.

For the remaining two days, you will eat approximately 500 to 600 calories.

The baseline of the calorie ingestion is 2,000 for women and 2,500 for men.

A few famous names swear by the diet including Jennifer Aniston and David Cameron.

These are some of the ways of how to manage the 5:2 diet plan.

Just remember carbs don't mix with your fasting days.

Experiment with Mealtime

- Test different eating times.

  It doesn't always have to be an early time of day when you aren't hungry.

  You can wait a bit longer if you wish.

- Change from eating three meals each day to two such as having brunch.

  It can combine the meals and save the calories.

Try having brunch around 11 am and dinner at 7 pm, or even a larger meal at 8 pm with your significant other.

Maximize the Flavoring and Minimize the Calories

- Soups are a respectable choice—also proven by research—because you remain full longer than just a modest serving of veggies on a plate.

- Flavor your foods with spices and herbs such as these—lemon juice or vinegar for salads or curry pastes or chili flakes in stews, baked beans, or soups.

- Go for the veggies and salads with smaller servings of fish, eggs, lean meat, or tofu.

Use Fresh Ingredients

- Not only are you eating better and healthier products, but also most fresh ingredients are less expensive.

  Search for seasonal produce for the most savings.

- Search for items such as a tomato that have ripened.

  These will make a yummy treat with a few of your special herbs and balsamic vinegar.

  You could also add it to some soup.

- During the winter months, experiment with butternut squash or parsnip—roasted—with low-fat feta—or in soup.

- Cut some peppers in half and stuff them with cream cheese, tuna, or similar ingredients and grill them.

You can add an egg to the mix for a taste challenge.

Food for the Fasting Days

- Berries and natural yogurt

- Plentiful veggie portions

- Baked or boiled eggs

- Low-calorie cup soups

- Other soups: vegetable, tomato, miso, cauliflower

- Lean mean or grilled fish

- Tea or black coffee

- Water (sparkling or still)

The 4:3 Diet Plan

Health benefits include asthma relief, reduction in heart arrhythmias, insulin resistance, menopausal hot flashes, seasonal allergies, and much more.

After twelve weeks of fasting using the 4:3 method diet plan, these are the results from a small study group:

- Fat mass reduction: 3.5 kg with no muscle mass changes

- Body weight reduction: Over 5 kg

- Increased LDL particle size

- Reduced blood levels: 20% reduction of triglycerides

- Leptin levels: 40% decreased

- Levels CRP: Reduced levels (inflammation marker in your body)

How the 4:3 Diet Plan is Different from the 5:2 Plan

The 5:2 intermittent fasting choices are much simpler than the 4:3 Plan because you are more restricted.

You will be intermittently fasting for three out of the seven days.

You should not eat processed/sugary/refined foods for four of the days.

If you do, your body will crave the supplementary fatty acids you need to thrive.

If you consume junk on those four days, you will defeat the purpose of the plan.

Just remember, not to over-indulge.

As you train your body by eating a well-planned diet; your body will adjust to the routine, and you won't feel as hungry.

The 4:3 Plan acclaims you skip the morning meal, and it recommends you check your weight daily.

However, this can be disheartening if your weight fluctuates.

A sample plan for the 4:3 method of weight loss is as follows:

- *Breakfast:* Eat nothing.

- *Lunch:* Leek, lentil, or chicken soup with a snack such as a small tangerine

- *Dinner:* A side salad using lemon juice as the dressing with some salt, pepper, or similar seasonings along with a small lean fillet of grilled chicken

- *Snacks:* Veggies or fruit

You can have a light breakfast if you enjoy a morning meal, but you will need to eliminate the snack during the day.

You can also skip lunch, and have a larger breakfast.

This is more challenging to follow than the 5:2 intermittent fasting plan because you have three days you can only consume 500 calories versus two days on the 5:2 diet.

Suggestions for the Fasting Days Using the 4:3 Method

- Drink an abundance of water.

- Drink coffee and tea for an additional boost.

- Consume a 400-calorie meal with a snack of 100 total calories.

- Chew sugar-free gum to fight the hunger spurts.

If you have a busy lifestyle, you can cheat once in a while with a low-calorie pre-packaged meal. (This is not a regular outlet.)

The point in both plans is to eat as much as you want and not feel deprived on the days you can eat normally—just do it in moderation, not over-indulgence.

Chapter 8: Tips and Simple Meal Plans

Simple Guidelines to Follow for Fasting

Stay in Control: Depending on which method you choose for your intermittent fasting routine, you need to ask the question if you can follow the crucial diet plans involved to keep your food intake at proper levels.

If you are attempting to achieve a 500-calorie debit daily, you have to keep your appetite under control, because a single missed meal won't provide a generous window for the next meal.

Keep a Calorie Tally Record: You must keep an accurate record of your calorie intake because if you are not careful, you can easily overeat at mealtime.

If your goal is to work off more calories than you consume to lose the one pound of weight you want to lose each week.

Stay with the Chosen Plan: You need to get into the habit of setting a regular schedule for your fasting plan.

Once your body adjusts to the specific method, it will become confused if you try another plan.

For example, if you are on the 5:2 plan and switch to the 16:8 plan, your body will stop the weight loss until it can readjust to the new plan.

You will lose valuable time by switching.

Consistency is essential for a successful fasting plan.

Breakfasts and Snacks

While you are attempting to lose weight on the intermittent fasting plan, you should not feel the need to be hungry no matter which of the procedures you decide to use.

Some of the recipes call for grams which need to be converted to ounces.

Use this <u>handy chart</u> to calculate the amounts.

This chapter is dedicated to some of the meals you can use.

Each menu plan has a calorie count within the recipe.

Breakfast

Porridge

89 Calories: 25 g Porridge oats
10 Calories: ½ teaspoon honey
0 Calories: Water and Cinnamon

Tips:
Instead of milk, use some water to reduce the calorie count. For some additional flavor add just a pinch of cinnamon. You can also improve the meal with a few nuts if you add the calories to your plan.

Toast and Beans

55 Calories: 1 slice whole- meal bread (small loaf size)
42 Calories: 50 g Baked beans

For a quick and low-calorie choice, tempt your taste buds with this unique idea.

Fruity Breakfast Meals

Watermelon

The natural sugars are more beneficial than a cereal bar. 96 Calories: 300 g serving

Honey and Bananas

10 Calories: ½ teaspoon honey
89 Calories: 1 small banana

Apricots and Yogurt

68 Calories: Two chopped apricots and 25 g Greek yogurt (low-fat)

Apricots, Greek Fat-Free Yogurt, and Mixed Berries

- 24 Calories: 3 tablespoons Greek yogurt
- 17 Calories: 1 Apricot
- 19 Calories: 50 g Raspberries
- 16 Calories: 50 g Strawberries
- 20 Calories: 50 g Blackberries
- Total Calories: 96

Blend the ingredients for a yummy treat.

Greek Yogurt, Sultanas, & Almonds

- 24 Calories: 3 tablespoons Greek Yogurt (fat-free)
- 42 Calories: 1 tablespoon sultanas
- 28 Calories: 4 almonds (whole)
- Total Calorie Intake: 94

Blueberries, Kiwi, & Greek Yogurt

- 42 Calories: 1 kiwi (chopped)
- 29 Calories: Blueberries (50g)
- 24 Calories: 3 tablespoons yogurt

Total Intake: 95 Calories

Mix all the ingredients for a tasty meal.

Raspberry and Cranberry Smoothie

- 14 ounces/175 g raspberries
- 7 ounces cranberry juice
- 3 ounces natural yogurt
- Mint sprigs

For a quick and easy breakfast try this one packing 100 calories per serving.
Serves 4 to 6 people

Eggs for Breakfast

Plain Eggs

100 Calories: 1 large boiled egg
Add a slice of wheat toast with two small poached eggs for a 188-calorie delight.

Scrambled with Mushrooms

78 Calories: 1 medium egg
13 Calories: fresh chopped mushrooms (100 g)
Total Count: 91 Calories

Scramble the ingredients and enjoy!

Spinach Omelet

16 Calories: 60 g fresh spinach
78 Calories: 1 medium egg
Total Calorie Count: 94

Instructions
1. Simply, beat/whisk the egg and place in a frying pay.
2. When the bottom is cooked; add spinach to the top and grill.
3. If you want, you can add some herbs, salt, or pepper for additional flavoring.

Ham Omelet

19 Calories: 1 slice of ham/wafer sliced
78 Calories: 1 Egg (medium)

Prepare the ingredients as above.

Starchy Options

Bread with Honey

55 Calories: 1 slice bread (whole meal from a small loaf)
40 Calories: 2 teaspoons honey
Total: 95

Perfect Pancakes

2 eggs
1 1/3 cups milk (300 ml) 100 g all-purpose flour
Sunflower Oil

Instructions
Blend the ingredients, cook, and sprinkle with a splash of lemon juice.

114 Calories: Per serving

Total Servings: 4

Pancake Variation

2 whole eggs
1 ripe banana

Instructions
1. Simply blend the two ingredients until the bananas are completely mashed.
2. Gently grease a pan with a sprinkle of oil and add the batter.
3. Cook 20 to 30 seconds, flip them over and enjoy.

Calorie counts: 1 medium banana/118 g/105 calories
2 large eggs/100 g/156 calories

A total of 261 calories is not bad for these yummy delights!

In Advance: Fiber-Packed Cereal

If you have a busy lifestyle and always rush in the morning, consider making this tasty breakfast bowl. It will serve 18 meals at 124 calories each.

- 100 g All-bran

- 300 g jumbo oats

- 50 g golden linseed

- 25 g wheat germ

- 140 g ready-to-eat apricots (chunked)

- 100 g dark raisins

Instructions
1. Blend all the ingredients.

2. Ahead of time break down each of the units and store in airtight containers.

3. To serve: Add milk and let it soak. Grate some unpeeled apple over it for a flavor delight.

Note: The cereal can be safely stored for two months in the airtight container.

Snacks

Snack time doesn't always have to be boring.

You can trick your mind by using the small plate.

Add some of these healthier choices to your intermittent fasting meal plan for weight loss.

You will also notice the 'not so healthy' choices are higher calorie content, but that is the advantage of planning your menu before you are hungry.

Each of these yummy delights will keep you going until lunchtime:

- 130 Calories: One square dark chocolate and a small banana

- 55 Calories: 10 g of 85% Dark chocolate

- 75 Calories: 3 Stuffed celery sticks with low-fat cottage cheese

- 96 Calories: 16 olives (green or black)

Epic Rios

- 90 Calories: 1 Cup Cherries

- 29 Calories: 100 g Honeydew melon

- 42 Calories: 2 Satsumas/tangerine (The Christmas Orange)

- 90 Calories: 3 thin slices Pineapple

- 61 Calories: 100 g Grapes/ OR 100 Calories: 30 grapes

- 42 Calories: Sun-Maid Mini Box of Raisins

- 90 Calories: 25 Pistachio nuts

- 74 Calories: 10 Salted peanuts

Each Item Counts as 100 Calories:

- 31 Asparagus Spears

- 9—5" Spears of Broccoli

- 16 ribs Celery

- 12 Raw Brussels Sprouts

- 28 Baby Carrots

- 82 Red Kidney Beans

- 60 Raw Green Beans

- 43 Boiled or Steamed Okra Pods

- 100 Radishes

- 20 Sun-Dried Tomatoes

- 22 Cloves Garlic

- 100 Raspberries

- 5 Dried Figs

- 6 Dried Apricots

- 8 Cashew Nuts

- 10 Pringles Chips

- 21 Pretzels Unsalted Minis

- 4 Sardines in Oil Drained

- 13 Large Boiled or Steamed Shrimp

- 15 pieces Dry-Roasted Cashew Halves

Tasty Beverages Too Good to Pass Up!

Starbucks Grande Skinny Iced Latte: 96 Calories

Avocado—Chocolate Milkshake: 169 Total Calories/2 servings

Simply blend and enjoy:

1 ½ cups skim milk
2 tablespoons each:

- Brown sugar

- Cocoa powder

½ ripe avocado
1 teaspoon vanilla extract

These are just a few of the tasty treats you can have in store for you while you are on the intermittent fasting diet plan.

There are many more for you to discover that will have you losing weight and toning those muscles to get fit in no time!

Conclusion

Thank you again for downloading *Intermittent Fasting: Lose Fat, Build Muscle and Get Fit*!

I hope it provided you with the understanding of the wide variety of options you have when it comes to intermittent fasting and how you can best mix and match to find the perfect solution for you.

Making the decision to alter your primary eating patterns is a major one, and it is important that you take the full weight of the decision into account before acting.

If you are convinced that you have what it takes to take full advantage of the benefits that intermittent fasting has to offer, then the next step is to stop reading, and to start fasting.

Choose the type of intermittent fasting that seems like the best fit for you and give it a try.

Try not to become discouraged if you don't receive immediate results.

Make an effort to find the one that's right for you.

Above all, don't rush, and remember, intermittent fasting is a marathon not a sprint, slow and steady will win the race.

Lastly, if you found this book useful in any way, a review on Amazon is always appreciated!

Bodybuilding
How to Build the Body of a Greek God

Table of Contents

presented is without assurance regarding its continued validity or interim quality.

Trademarks that mentioned are done without written consent and can in no way be considered an endorsement from the trademark holder.

Introduction

Congratulations on downloading your personal copy of *Bodybuilding: How to Build the Body of a Greek God.* Thank you for doing so.

These days, bodybuilding information is everywhere. Building toned and big bodies seem to be the norm, but is that really what we are looking for?

This book looks at the classic Greek God physique, one that is strong and capable but not overwhelmingly showy.

With big, clunky bodies becoming the norm for good physique these days, we need an alternative for normal people.

The Greek body is one that is built on hard work and military training, not focused on putting in hours of weight training at the gym every day. Instead, Greeks were hard working warriors and farmers and their bodies reflected that functionality.

The following chapters will discuss how to create a modern-day workout with focus on the old Greek ways of bodybuilding in order to build a healthy, strong body that is more than just a showpiece.

Here, we will discuss specific workouts and nutrition plans that will help get your ideal body.

You will discover how important maintaining an overall healthy lifestyle is in creating an ideal Greek body, and how rewarding maintaining your new physique will be to your mental, physical and social quality of life.

There are plenty of books on bodybuilding on the market, but none quite like this. Thanks again for choosing this one! Every effort was made to ensure it is full of as much useful information as possible. Please enjoy!

Chapter 1: Greek Bodies in Art: Drawings and Statues

In order to truly understand what we are striving for with a Greek physique, we must understand the history behind the ideal Greek body, as it is a rich and vibrant one.

First off, the Greek empire existed from 800BC to 146BC, about three thousand years ago. Even though it was so long ago, Greek culture is still influencing civilizations around the world, including in the realm of health and fitness.

A major theme in Greek art throughout the centuries has been good order and form. The goal with any piece of art is to draw the eye and keep it by presenting something that makes sense to the eye and to the brain.

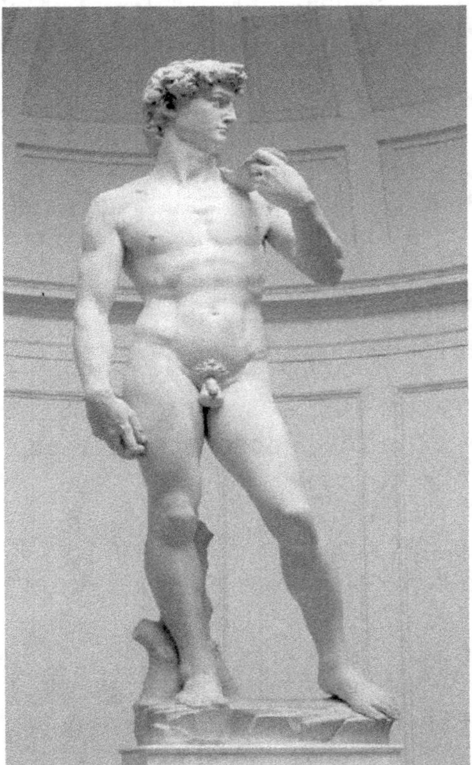

By using subjects that have perfect proportion will keep the eye looking, constantly drawn to the figure. These concepts have reflected into the work of well to do modern artists.

Creating a human form that is ideal and pleasing to the eye to keep people looking was the main focus.

The Greek body is considered an ideal standard for a number of reasons, one being the reputation of the Greeks to be a strong and conquering society.

The David, by Michelangelo

While their capital was in the Greece we know today, its empire reached through the modern day middle east.

Their citizens were considered the most fearsome warriors of the time, and war was glorified.

The strong and pioneering soldiers' body became typecast as the ideal Greek.

What is interesting and often forgotten in modern society is that the Greeks manufactured these ideal images in the likeness of Gods in which they have never actually met.

Just like in all religions, the idea of God is just that, an idea.

We have not seen this figure, but the human mind needs to put an image to the likeness.

The Greeks did just that. Their renderings of Gods and superhuman figures were not out of reality, but out of imagination.

Yes, the figure is generally the same, but lives up to the impossible standards of pure imagination.

These days, our standards are created by Photoshop, an ideal image rendered by the artist that is not a true reflection of reality.

Just like ancient Greeks, we try to live up to these standards unsuccessfully, perhaps because we are not immortal, and cannot dream to be.

We can dream of a perfect form but in nature, that doesn't exist. Sure, nature follows the Golden Rule often, but there are always imperfections.

The Greeks also established the Olympics. They created games in which they could showcase the strength and stamina of their people, something that could not be done with a less than ideal body.

While the focus was on winning sporting events, it also showcased the beauty and power of their ideal bodies.

The first Olympics was held in honor of Zeus, the most respected of their twelve Gods. Interestingly, nudity was common at the games, further showcasing the able bodies of participants.

The belief system of ancient Greece also brought rise to the idealistic body.

In Greek mythology, a total of fourteen Gods exist, all of which have their own strengths.

Zeus was the most powerful, the god of thunder and sky and of others, like Hades, the god of the underworld and Apollo, the god of the sun, among others.

What all of the male Greek gods had in common was their physique.

Regardless of their power and personal strength, their bodies were portrayed in just about the same way, following the natural form of the Golden Rule, a ratio that is most physically appealing to the eye.

Greek art always depicted the Gods as perfect creatures, who existed in a form that is in great proportion.

Some of the most famous artworks and sculptures were created during the classical period of Greece, between about 500 and 300BC.

This period of time has influenced the Roman Empire, and has had the most lasting impression through art and civilization surviving worldwide in modern times.

This is also the period in which Greek artists did their best work to recreate the ideal human form, thought to be a direct liking to the bodies of the Gods.

During this time, the proper ratios of the human body were extensively studied. The Greeks were so obsessed with the ideal human form that they were one of the first civilizations to quantify proper ratios of waist to height, waist and shoulder breadth and much more.

We will discuss these ratios in more detail in the next chapter.

Famous works of art, like Discobolus, a statue of the discus thrower are very iconic in that they show the Greek body in action.

We must remember that the Olympics originated in ancient Greece, and their contenders were the best of the best.

Their bodies were hard and strong, and able to carry out all of the games, including throwing the discus.

This sculpture shows the range of motion, the development of muscle and brute strength required to be an ideal figure.

Another popular Greek sculpture is The David, created by Michelangelo in the Renaissance period.

This sculpture is a work of art that cannot be compared to any other.

It depicts a young man of stellar form simply standing there, at about seventeen feet tall. With a coy smile and unwitting attitude, he simply is in all his glory; a Greek man. The musculature and details of the body show a man in his true, perfect form.

Speaking of Michelangelo, he is also responsible for his works in the Sistine Chapel in Vatican City.

His painting on the ceiling, The Creation of Adam is one of the most famous pieces of art ever created.

This iconic image shows the moment when God first creates Adam, the first human.

It shows the two touching fingers of their outstretched arms.

The bodies of both Adam and God are shown in ideal proportions, typical for Greek art.

We can see the purity of both figures because they have been painted in a way that depicts a flawless body; something to be attained.

Interestingly, the bodies of ancient Greek women and their goddesses are idealized in a much different way than we see in modern times.

Our current standard of beauty says that women should be stick thin yet muscular.

Looking at Greek art, we cannot compare these modern standards to the influences from ancient Greece. In fact, women are idolized as slender yet not stick thin.

They are in proper proportion with their waists more slender than their hips, yet hips were large and showed the ability to bear children, something that was much more important in ancient Greece.

There were no chiseled female chins or emphasis on rock hard abs. It was a much different, more lenient time for women, as their primary role was to be child bearer and caregiver, not like our modern CrossFit warriors.

Similarly, the standard for the male physique has changed as well.

There was a major shift in the late twentieth century that morphed the ideal male figure into that of a superhero.

His muscles must be big and strong, regardless of function. He would often look to topple over as his torso and upper body would be much larger than his lower half.

Think of modern day bodybuilders and men who use steroids to gain mass, yet function isn't always there.

This is so far against the ideal, functional warrior body of the Greek gods.

These days, we have traded function for "gym muscles", those that can bench press three hundred pounds but don't have the functionality to shovel manure in the garden or deadlift boxes in a warehouse.

The Greeks prided their ideal bodies on the ability to fight in wars, maintain their properties and provide food for their families.

They did not have modern day tools and equipment to do the heavy lifting, they did it with brute strength and agility.

Chapter 2: Proportions of Greek Gods

Ancient Greeks took their physiques very seriously.

It was considered a sign of strength, power and virility to maintain a certain physique.

This was modeled after the perfection of Greek Gods, who were immortal and strong.

They even went as far as to consider specific measurements desirable.

 Much like bodybuilders today, Greeks were obsessed with obtaining the perfect body.

Overall, the perfect Greek body was one that was functional and strong.

Greece was often in war, and needed healthy, strong fighters to maintain their armies and fight their enemies.

The Greeks were warriors, and it was necessary to have a strong, functional figure to even have a fighting chance against their enemies.

Men trained to be powerful, agile and fast in order to defeat their enemies.

Good fighters were naturally lean, carrying very little fat. They also had strong upper bodies but did not have overly developed arm muscles like current day bodybuilders.

They needed to be able to travel on foot to new fields of battle.

Once they got there, they could not take a break, they needed to fight.

Stamina was a huge part of training. Being able to run long distances then not keel over upon arrival was an absolute must.

Those who could not keep up would be left behind and would be the first to die in the event of battle.

Men trained to survive, not just to look good naked.

These days, there are fewer opportunities to fight in battle, and even our current army has vehicles to move people around and sophisticated weaponry to prevent hand to hand combat.

The Greeks were often face-to-face with their enemies, wielding swords and shields. They needed brute strength to use them and not get tired out easily.

Even men who did not fight in the Greek military were strong.

Those who were not fighting were farmers and workers who spent their day sowing fields and bailing hay.

These men could lift items over their heads while pulling on their livestock. There rarely were situations in which they would need to bench press weights. Instead, they had functional strengths, the kind that gets real work done.

The ideal measurements of a strong working man were as follows: for the bicep, 16.4 inches in diameter.

As compared to modern bodybuilding, this is puny.

The ideal neck is 16.8 inches in diameter, the chest 45.5-inch diameter and forearms should be 13.2 inches in diameter.

This seems like quite a specific ratio to shoot for, and if you were a Greek, reaching these goals was a matter of day to day living.

As for the lower body, Greeks had naturally strong and muscular legs, ones that could run long distances, be agile enough to evade enemies, and strong enough to wrangle livestock and do daily chores.

Again, it is all about function. A perfect thigh is 24.1 inches in diameter and the calf 15.5 inches.

We must not forget that Greeks also had a very strong core.

The abdomen and back are the muscles at the center of every movement. They swing arms and legs in controlled, exact movements. They lift heavy items, including fallen comrades in battle.

These muscles were slender and not overbuilt.

A perfect waist is 31.9 inches, and hips 38.7 inches.

Hearing about these perfect measurements may seem like a turn-off.

How on earth is an everyday person able to meet these perfect standards.

Truthfully, it is a matter of luck when it comes to bone structure that allows your hips to measure 38.7 inches, regardless of fat. Some men are just bigger.

If you feel like this book is no longer for you just based on these measurements alone, don't get discouraged.

Honestly, it will be a miracle to attain and maintain these perfect numbers, so don't focus so much on it.

Instead, we must consider the Golden Ratio, a number that is much simpler to understand.

Rather than focusing on reaching a certain inch, we must look at the overall proportion within your measurements.

A simple equation can get us there: $(A+B)/A = A/B$.

The perfect ratio is 1:1.618.

This is a much more manageable number to work with and can be used to compare all areas of your physique.

The Golden Ratio is actually found everywhere in the natural world, which is why it is so attractive and pleasing to the eye.

The Fibonacci sequence was developed by an Italian Mathematician named Leonardo Pisano in the middle ages.

By definition it is a sequence of numbers that are the sum of the two preceding numbers.

For example, if 1 and 2 are the first two numbers, three, and the sum of one and two would be the third, and five would be the fourth.

In nature, the Fibonacci sequence is all over.

A good example is tree branches.

The top of a tree fans out in a pattern in which the diameter of the tree follows this equation.

Flowers are the same way with their petals, and the seeds in the center of flowers, specifically sunflowers, make a spiral pattern that fits the equation perfectly.

It is only natural then that the human body also follows this natural pattern.

What we see as the perfect human figure is the tapering of the body from shoulders to waist in the Fibonacci sequence.

When it comes to human attraction, men who fit this ratio are considered scientifically more attractive to women.

The human face also follows this ratio. Ideal facial features should be aligned in a way that follows the natural order, and faces that fit this well are considered the most attractive.

Faces of animals are unconsciously judged using the same standards.

There are some more ratios to consider if perfection is what you're after.

Overall, your waist circumference should be 40-50% of your height, with ideal leaning more toward your height.

So, if you are six feet tall, or 72 inches, your ideal waist size is 36 inches.

Knowing your ideal waist size can help you determine your ideal shoulder size as well.

Use the Golden Ratio by multiplying your waist size times 1.618 to get 58 inches.

If your neck size is important as well, ideally it will measure about half of your waist size.

Your chest should also be 1.25 times your waist.

Properly proportion your lower half based on your upper body.

Your calves should measure about the same as your biceps. Remember to measure both at the largest section.

Your thighs should be strong yet slender, about .75 times the circumference of your waist.

To put it into perspective, the ideal body is described as one with broad shoulders, strong but not overly muscular arms.

The chest should be strong, tapering down to a slim, yet muscular core. The legs should be muscular as well, but lean.

This body is meant to work, and muscles are not meant to be shown off.

In clothes, a Greek body looks slender but toned.

There should be no bulging muscles trying to escape your tee shirt.

Wearing tighter clothing will help show off your new physique, but won't be steroid gaudy.

Your muscles should be understated, but the real magic comes out when you hit the beach.

Proper measurement is very important here, especially if you are taking these numbers to heart quite literally.

Measure your waist at the smallest part of your abdomen, just above the belly button.

Your natural waist hints in just a bit, and may not be exactly where your pants fall, although it should be pretty close, unless you like saggy pants.

Make sure to use a proper measurement technique as well. Use a cloth measuring tape that is typically used for sewing.

The flexibility of the tape will give you a more accurate number.

Also, have a friend help you, especially when it comes to measuring arms and legs. Stay relaxed and measure everything as is. You are not measuring the girth of your muscle when flexed, you want the look while relaxed.

Remember that there are certain features about ourselves that we cannot change.

Things dictated by our genetics, like the shape of our faces or the proportions of our bone structures cannot be meddled with (unless you are considering plastic surgery).

What we can do is use good nutrition and targeted workouts to do the best we can to manipulate muscle tone and percent body fat.

Use these measurements as a benchmark in order to guide your workout strategy, not as strict goal number.

Most likely, you will never meet these strict numbers exactly, so striving for it is a waste of time.

Instead, you want to enjoy your great new physique by showing it off, not by measuring yourself and obsessing about the numbers on a daily basis.

Still, in order to determine if your workout and diet program is working, keep track of your numbers monthly.

Keep the measurements as a guideline to make changes to your workouts as necessary.

Chapter 3: How Hollywood Portrays Greek Gods

While lots of things have changed since ancient Greece, our general physique and body make up has not.

It is possible to achieve the same look with some hard work. We have proof this is possible because of the work of many actors who have achieved the Greek body style to portray them in movies.

Remember that the goal is to have a body that is strong yet functionally useful, that's it. Everything else is just for show.

We have seen actors like Brad Pitt transform themselves into godlike forms for movies like Troy, in which he literally depicted a deity on earth, Achilles.

In the movie and in literature, Achilles is a fierce warrior who cannot be defeated.

His strength and agility are unmatched by any other fighter, and he is feared by all. Of course, as the story goes, he is eventually taken down by his only weakness, his heel.

As an arrow strikes his heel in the story, Achilles is killed. In the movie, it takes a few more to the chest to seem more realistic.

If we pick apart Brad Pitt's physique in this movie, we do not see body builder muscles. Instead, his muscles are there, toned, but understated.

His midsection is long and lean with strong, well-chiseled arms and legs. His muscles are not bulging, yet he is able to move quickly, defeating his enemies while swinging his sword and ducking arrows.

While movie magic certainly plays a role in the overall success of his character, proper training and exercise can help the average person look like our friend Brad Pitt.

Remember that in order to be Achilles, it will take some godly intervention and some serious combat training, but we can at least work on the look.

Another great Brad Pitt body movie is Fight Club.

This 1999 gem has Brad Pitt as Tyler Durden, a founding member of an underground fighting ring in which members battle each other with gloves off, no rules action.

Although traditional Greek warfare is out the window here, Brad Pitt carries the same physique as his character in Troy.

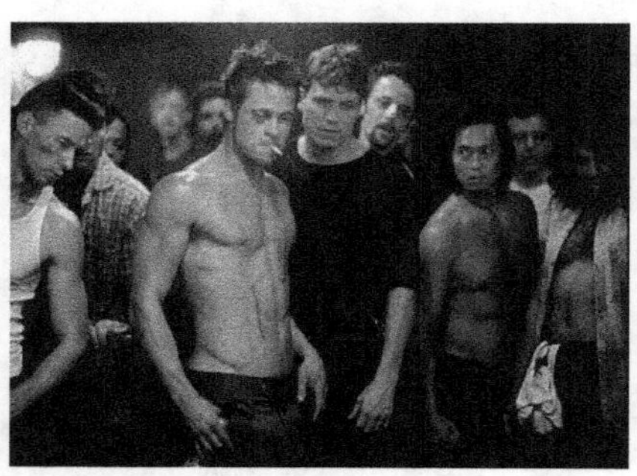

He is long, lean and muscular. More importantly, he is quick and smart, able to duck blows and take down his adversaries.

What is different in this movie is how cut he looks compared to Achilles in Troy.

Tyler Durden is meant to look scrappy, squirrely and a little bit crazy.

His face is chiseled, while a bit gaunt. He has very little fat, and his muscles are more defined.

Brad Pitt, Fight Club It is implied that his body is there to destroy others, and little else.

While there are many Greek movies out, like Troy, 300 and many of the genre, there are also lots of superhero movies out lately.

We must make the distinction between the typical Greek God body and the Superhero body.

While both are strong and muscular, the superhero body is more of a likeness to the modern bodybuilder.

Bodybuilding took hold in the 1940s, and made the body more of a spectacle than ever before.

While chiseled bodies were formerly used for work, the boundaries had been pushed to show just how big muscles could get.

The upper body was usually the biggest, while maintaining a tiny waist. The idea of proper Greek proportions was totally out the window.

Bodybuilding competitions quickly took off, with top contenders having very large, sometimes steroid induced pecs and biceps with tiny, almost womanlike waists.

The addition of orange spray tan and baby oil was simply a bonus.

While a bit exaggerated, the superhero model body took after these images of bodybuilders.

These days, Marvel and other comic book giants have made movies of just about every superhero out there.

Superman and Thor are gracing the covers of DVDs all over the world.

Their upper bodies are large and in charge, almost carrying too much muscle to be any help.

It's a good thing superhuman strength is built into their job description.

Chris Hemsworth plays Thor in the most recent Avengers series and has a typical superhero build.

While his muscle and tone is something to be admired, the look is very different from the Greek ideal, and not what we are going for here.

Cartoon depictions of superheroes are even more exaggerated.

Take a look at the character Metroman in the Dreamworks movie Megamind. His character has a huge upper body and puny waist and legs.

Yes, it's a cartoon but is also a spoof on the modern day overbuilt upper body.

Chapter 4: Get Muscles of a Greek God

Getting the body of a Greek God may actually be easier and more productive than you think.

Remember that ancient Greek ideal bodies were that of functional human beings.

These people worked hard every day, training for battle as warriors or growing crops to feed their families.

They were building muscle by doing physical labor, not putting in reps at the gym. They certainly weren't doing it hiding behind a computer screen.

In order to build a workout routine, we must consider exactly what the Greeks were doing to obtain these bodies naturally and transform that into something we can do at home or at the gym in this modern era.

Several companies exist that purposely (or not) tailor routines that build strength through functional exercise. Perhaps the most popular right now is CrossFit.

Consider what kinds of exercises are done at CrossFit.

It centers around strength training with real life objects like tires.

Kettlebells are good representations of rocks that a Greek would have been hurling out of their garden.

The tires can represent just about anything heavy around their property that needed moving.

Remember that there was no heavy equipment to move large objects, just brute strength and the help of a few neighbors.

CrossFit also combines cardio exercise with weight training, which better mimics a real life work or war situation that a Greek may have been exposed to.

There are hardly any activities that involve only lifting, which is why typical lifting routines at the gym may be doing little for you.

While we will discuss cardio in more detail in the next chapter, just remember that it needs to be integrated into your routine for the best and fastest results.

That being said, a new trend is making it into the fitness world lately.

High intensity interval training, or HIIT for short, combines small bursts of intense cardio activity with weight training.

The result burns fat and builds muscle while saving time.

Many workouts exist online and in fitness centers everywhere.

When it comes to specific weight training, we need to think about what sets of muscles are used the most.

That is actually a trick question, because a well-rounded functional body uses all of the muscles equally.

Traditional bodybuilding has gotten us too focused on hitting the main ones, alternating between arm day and leg day, when in fact, we should be incorporating movements that incorporate all muscle groups in any given workout.

Your body knows how to use all of its strength at once to get the job done, and does not leave the arm muscles to lift something exclusively.

The back and legs help carry the weight. If you were to lift a bag of grass seed above your head while working in the yard, would you exclusively use your arms or would you distribute the weight evenly over your body?

While the Greeks had it figured out, we must find a way to tailor a workout routine to modern times.

Unless you have a physically strenuous job or have resources to work out outside every day of the year, this routine so far does not seem very feasible.

Instead, we need to modify the routine to work in a gym setting, something most of us are familiar with.

The key to the Greek workout routine is moderate weight strength training to build firm and functional muscles.

Making your goal to lift as much weight as humanly possible will get you a superhero style body.

If that's what you are going for, great, but maybe you should be reading another book.

The goal here is to build functional strength without overdoing it.

The good news is, you don't need to spend countless hours at the gym to get a great body, just smart, targeted exercises.

Weight training in the gym no longer means hitting every machine. Think about your current routine and every individual exercise that you do.

As you complete each motion, can you think of a way that you could carry out the same motion in real life?

For example, how often are you, or your Greek counterpart required to deadlift over a hundred pounds?

While a few instances may exist, their bodies are not built to do that on a regular basis because it just isn't necessary.

Same with bicep curls. That is a very specific movement that only targets one muscle. Most likely, they are working their biceps and the rest of their arm muscles at the same time, not individually.

Just looking at the ideal Greek figure, we can tell that they were not bench pressing excessive weight, as their chests were defined but not huge.

While using weight machines and free weights can mimic functional exercise, it can only come so far.

This is why interval training, and doing activities that combine muscle training with real life situations is so important.

There were no gyms in ancient Greece, and nobody was counting reps. That is a modern day institution that does not translate.

Instead, focus your time on taking classes that combine lots of disciplines, and things that the Greeks would likely be doing.

Greek warriors would practice fighting. They wrestled, boxed, and practiced with swords.

Today, we can recreate some of this with kickboxing classes and martial arts training. Of course, the Olympics were founded around the javelin, discus and other common track and field exercises.

Get involved with local teams to practice your long jump and throwing skills. You will be ready to battle the Persians in no time.

The good old calisthenics your grandfather used to do are useful too.

Use body weight exercises like sit ups, pushups and planks to build a strong core.

This variety of body weight exercises combines repetition of movement to increase muscle tone, induce cardio exercise and improve flexibility.

The best part is, these routines can be done just about anywhere and don't require any equipment.

If financial restrictions are keeping you out of the gym, hit the floor and get to some crunches and pushups. Use sturdy tree limbs or buy a pull up bar to practice pull ups.

The idea behind calisthenics is body weight training, and by nature does not require too much equipment or skill.

If working out is new to you and committing to bulky equipment or buying a gym membership isn't for you, calisthenics is.

The best way to go about a calisthenics routine is to pick a variety of exercises to do in a circuit.

Each exercise should focus on a different muscle group and be done to near exhaustion.

For example, choose to do pushups until your arms get a bit shaky, then quickly move on to an abdominal routine.

Do something that works for each muscle group individually until everything has been touched.

In the end, your heart should be pumping hard to get blood to all of your muscles, and you will begin to tone up and slim down.

If you do choose to work outside the gym, either for convenience, monetary reasons or just a change of scenery, channel your inner Greek god.

Particularly, Poseidon, the God of the sea, did a lot of swimming.

Regular workouts in the pool or local lake will work all of your muscles at once, and the resistance of the water creates just enough pull to really cut and define your body without looking like a gym lunk.

Alternate different types of swimming strokes. Do the breaststroke, which focuses mainly on the chest and backstroke for your back.

Your legs will pretty much be kicking the whole time but alternate between a normal kick and a frog kick to work different muscle groups.

As you get outside, think of the ancient Greek military climbing the Pindus Mountains to reach their enemies.

Those guys were climbing day and night, so a craggy hillside hike will certainly help define those leg muscles while also building cardio stamina.

Gardening, working with animals and construction are other great ways to build your physique.

If you are really dedicated, trade your desk job for a building career. Or, if you like your cushy position, just volunteer with a home building service on weekends.

Starting a garden on your property is much more than planting seeds. It is tilling up the soil, hoeing and clearing weeds and lifting all sorts of tools.

It requires time every couple of days to keep on top of things, so this is a great way to build some accountability into your routine.

Plus, the vegetables you grow will make a great addition to your new Greek style diet, which we will talk more about later.

How do you measure your success?

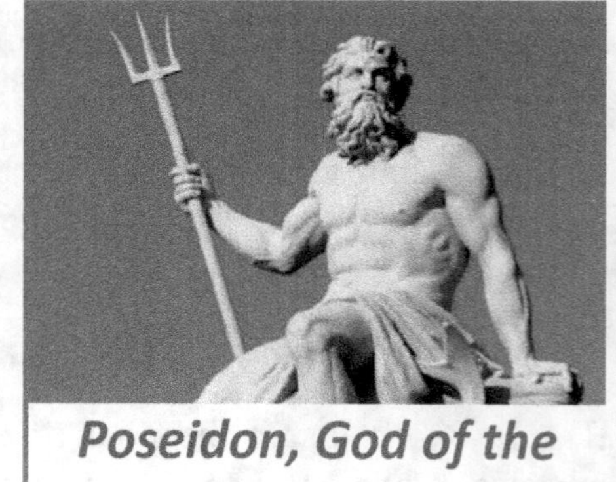

Poseidon, God of the Sea

Any bodybuilding website will tell you that signs of progress come with increased tolerance for weight and number of reps.

But we're not going for a superhero, are we?

Your measure for success should come with functional strength.

Find ways to measure your success in real life like a Greek would.

Volunteer to help your friend move heavy furniture. Volunteer with a local construction company and haul some cement blocks.

Regularly test your strength in real life situations.

Following a regular routine of functional strength training should create better ability to lift heavy objects, move them in awkward positions, and give you the stamina to keep going.

To get started, measure your baseline. Do an activity that you know will give you some physical challenge.

Try entering an obstacle course event or just going to a CrossFit class.

Focus on how your muscles feel during and after the exercise.

Are they burning or giving out? This means you have work to do.

On the ancient battlefield, you would already be dead.

Think of your training as a life and death situation, because you never actually know when you may need strength and stamina to save your own life or that of another.

Hopefully, that gives you a little more motivation as well.

After you begin training, do that baseline activity again, and see how you compare.

Hopefully, your muscles will be better able to handle the hell you are putting them through.

Remember that a good workout is always one that challenges you, so don't make your goal finishing with little effort.

This just means that it is time to step it up and rise to a more difficult baseline.

In the course of your new workout regimen, keep the Greek workout philosophy in mind.

There are no workouts, just work.

Greeks exercised and worked their muscles to get things done.

With the invention of computers and heavy equipment to do work in modern times, chances to get this type of exercise are few and far between unless you seek them out.

Tailor your workouts to real life situations, particularly ones that you will encounter in the future.

As you do this, your muscles will lean out and change, with little additional effort and extra reps at the gym.

If you have no idea where to get started, check out Chapter 6 for an 8-week example guide to start your workouts.

Chapter 5: Cutting Fat With Cardio

Those muscles mean nothing if they are hiding behind a layer of fat.

We have talked a lot about muscle tone for an ideal body, but fat plays a major role as well.

You will recall those perfect proportions we discussed earlier in the book.

Adding fat to any area of the body will change your ratios.

Everybody carries weight a little differently, leading to a couple of extra inches here and there.

Nobody ever gains weight evenly across the whole thing.

Some will have a larger belly, larger butt or carry it all in the thighs.

It is insane to ask for zero percent body fat, as fat is actually necessary for life.

It cushions your vital organs and is necessary as part of your skin and brain makeup.

We cannot eliminate it completely, but we can make sure it stays in check and where we want it.

Tone and strengthen all you want, they will not be seen unless you can melt some of the fat that cushions the muscle.

The only surefire way to burn fat in the body is with cardiovascular exercise.

As we have learned from Greek art, the ideal body was toned and taught, not loose and flabby.

If that is your baseline, don't worry, there are lots we can do to fix it.

The current thinking is that the ideal Greek body was about 10% fat, a far cry from the baseline fat level of 25-30% in today's society.

Aerobic exercise, by definition, is anything that uses oxygen to burn energy.

Many types of exercise create this result, but weight lifting is not one of them.

Weight lifting is anaerobic activity, which does not require the use of oxygen to make energy.

To make it simple, exercises that use oxygen are those that make you out of breath, like running or swimming.

Sure, muscles can be built with these exercises as well, but the main purpose for cardio activity is to work the heart muscle and to burn fat.

The heart is literally at the heart of all exercises, pumping blood full of fresh oxygen to cells and muscles in order to keep the movement going.

A strong heart is an absolute necessity to carry out all activities, and it is important that we keep it healthy.

Working out the heart gives us more stamina over time.

Regular exercise strengthens the heart, making it more efficient at pumping oxygen to muscles, which is required for the overall stamina of muscles in the arms and legs.

Working this muscle for an ancient Greek could have been a matter of life and death.

A warrior that was out of shape would quickly lose to an enemy who was in peak performance, simply out of basic health.

If fat is what you're after, aerobic exercise is your key to success.

The body is a complicated machine that runs on several types of fuel.

The body prefers to use energy from carbohydrates as a primary source of fuel.

Carbohydrates are things like pasta, bread and other simple sugars that can be easily be broken down for energy.

As we eat, the body uses a majority of the energy right away, and whatever it doesn't need is stored as fat for future use.

Often times, we eat more than our bodies need at any given time, and lots of food becomes stored as fat.

A few very common misconceptions occur here.

It isn't just excess fat that gets stored as fat. Any excess calories, whether from fat, carbohydrate or protein will be converted and stored as fat, no questions asked.

The body's metabolism is meant to help us survive, and therefore has the ability to keep anything and everything it doesn't need to fit its urgent needs.

It is meant to be kept for times when food is not available.

In this day and age, excess food is a problem not lack of food, for most people.

During the normal course of the day, the body will burn simple sugars it gets from food to perform normal tasks.

A small amount of these sugars are stored in the liver to use for the remainder of the day.

This includes simple walks around the office, getting lunches ready, cleaning the house and so on.

It is only when this supply in the liver runs out that the body must tap into additional resources for energy. This is where aerobic activity really shines.

During high-intensity exercises like running, or even walking long distances, the liver's supply of sugar is quickly depleted, and the body must pull stored energy from fat cells to fuel the body.

During these times, fat is the main source of energy, and will be until the body is replenished with simple sugars from the diet.

It is during these periods that we need to take advantage of the body's natural metabolism to burn fat for us.

The jury is really out on the timing of meals for fat loss.

Based on this theory, one would assume that exercising on an empty stomach would cause the liver stores to deplete much quicker, putting us in a fat burning mode.

However, we know that eating after a workout will quickly stop fat burning and cause us to go back to burning sugar.

While this all seems ideal, we do need to eat at some point, and the liver will have sugars stored no matter what.

What we do know is that exercising on an empty stomach leads to less energy and intensity during the workout, leading to less calorie burn.

Therefore, it is a good idea to fuel up before a workout, but not to overdo it. We will get more into the science of meal timing in the following chapters.

Cardiovascular exercise burns calories more efficiently than weight training, and weight loss in its simplest terms means burning more calories than you consume.

Not to mention that you are still working some muscles while you run or swim, and muscles require more energy to maintain than fat cells, naturally increasing your body's energy needs for the day.

The body continues to burn fat after a cardio workout is over as well, so it is advantageous to wait about half an hour after exercise to eat.

This is said with a word of caution, as people with health conditions like diabetes need to be vigilant of hypoglycemia, where their blood sugar drops dangerously low.

For the typical individual, showering and dressing after a workout is likely long enough to go before having a quick snack.

Beginning an aerobic routine can be a bit daunting, but getting started with simple steps can get even the most dedicated couch potato into shape.

First, you must determine your baseline level.

If just walking to the mailbox makes you feel winded, you will need to take it slow.

If you are reading this book, we would assume your baseline is a bit higher than that. But perhaps you are a dedicated walker and running makes you feel light-headed and nauseous.

Building up cardio stamina is just like weight training. You need to start small and increase your intensity to build upon your success.

Just as you might start with a five-pound weight with your bicep curls, start with just a few minutes at a light jog during your walk.

Increase your heart rate to a safe level, then bring it back down to baseline.

In general, your pace should allow you to sing or carry on a conversation with your partner as you walk or jog.

If you are so winded that you could not do either, your pace is too fast.

It is important to push yourself past your baseline in order to increase your stamina and calorie burning potential, it is the only way to make improvements.

Just like you would push your muscles until they become a bit shaky, you must get yourself a little out of breath to get that heart working and building muscle memory.

Burning fat is not just about intensity. In fact, studies have shown that fat is burned more efficiently at moderate intensity exercise levels.

Working out too fiercely and getting your heart pumping too hard actually works against you.

Remember that the heart's primary job during cardio exercise is delivering oxygen to your muscles for stamina.

If your muscles work too hard and the oxygen cannot get there, the body works in anaerobic mode, burning sugars in the muscle for fuel.

Both aerobic and anaerobic exercises burn energy, but anaerobic exercise produces lactic acid, which makes muscles feel tired and fatigued, increasing the need for recovery time.

Staying within a relatively safe cardio routine will ensure that you build the stamina you need to exercise more efficiently, but will help in recovery time by not exhausting muscles with lactic acid.

Overall, any extra exercise you do will help burn fat and help you reach your goals.

To start a routine, determine your baseline, just as you would with weight training.

Depending on your time schedule, either add a few minutes each day to your cardio workout or increase the intensity.

Adding interval sprints or aiming to walk or jog just a bit faster will slowly increase your stamina and overall ability.

As your heart and lung strength improve, you will likely see this overlap and make daily tasks that were once difficult a whole lot easier.

Being consistent with cardiovascular training is necessary as well.

You can't work out for a week and expect to maintain the same stamina a month later if you don't continue your routine.

The body declines very quickly into couch potato status if it is not regularly worked, so whatever activity you decide to fit into your daily routine, make sure it is manageable, and something you have time to do on a regular basis.

From a health standpoint, exercise is pushed at us from every angle and is a necessary part of good health.

It would be a good idea to rearrange your priorities a bit to put your exercise routine and your overall health at the top of your list.

After all, you can't get everything else you need to do done unless your body is around to do it.

Certainly, we did not mean to skirt past the issue of sugars and calories coming in from the diet.

Surely, a proper diet routine must fit in here somewhere? Indeed it does, so much so that it gets its own chapter.

Learn more about fueling your workouts and reducing fat buildup through diet in Chapter 9.

Chapter 6: Your 8-Week Weight Training Guide

Everybody will have a different starting point, so it is important to tailor this routine to your specific fitness level.

The guide that follows starts with one week of half hour workouts that are meant to progress as weeks go on.

If you feel that starting with shorter workouts is more feasible for your current level, go ahead and cut it in half to start.

The idea is to progress and get stronger based on your baseline, not everyone else's.

Your goal is to get stronger than you are now, not to compete with others.

Also, these exercises are meant to work out all muscle groups.

If former injuries or disabilities make any of these routines dangerous or painful, modify them to preserve your function.

Remember that even Achilles had a weak ankle, so if you do too, don't do exercises that aggravate the problem.

You will notice that there are only workouts scheduled six days a week.

Every good Greek knows that a day of rest and recovery is a key to a healthy body.

Make sure to relax at least one day a week to allow your muscles to fully repair.

Overworking muscles can lead to decreased performance over time, lethargy and even injury.

Who needs that?

All weight training and weight bearing exercises are meant to be done slowly.

The faster you try to complete the exercise, the less energy is used because momentum is used instead of muscle strength.

Take your time and really put in the work.

Never lock elbows or knees, keep the pressure on your muscles to hold up your weight.

Being a true Greek means incorporating more real life exercises as well.

This routine can be used to get a good baseline going, but be sure to incorporate exercises like hiking, swimming, and other more strenuous activities a few times a week for best results.

Week One: Determine your baseline and warm up

This first week should be dedicated to finding out where you stand physically.

Test your overall strength, agility and flexibility with these exercises.

Get started with this set of exercises, which should take about half an hour once you get going.

These exercises are easy to complete and can be done anywhere.

Should you be traveling or in a situation where you have less time or ability to get to the gym, these exercises can be done.

Monday, Wednesday, Friday

•	10-minute jog/treadmill- outside or in place, to increase the heart rate.

•	20 sit ups x 3 sets- may do more if your baseline fitness level is high. Do as many as possible until your muscles begin to tremble.

- 1-minute jog in place to return heart rate to cardio level.

- 20 pushups x 3 sets- do full pushups or on knees per baseline strength. Again, do more if your baseline is higher.

- 20 pull ups x 3 sets- keep back straight, good posture, do not let elbows lock at the bottom.

- 1-minute jumping jacks in place to return heart rate to cardio level.

- 20 squats x 3 sets- no weights required. Weight should be centered on the heel of the foot, stretching down so upper thigh is parallel to the ground.

- 1-minute jog in place to return heart rate to cardio level.

- 30-second plank x 3 sets- keep back straight, complete on elbows or hands. For extra workout, lift feet off the ground a few inches, alternating feet. This will increase muscle strength in the back and butt.

- 1-minute jog in place to return heart rate to cardio level.

- Stretch and cooldown- stretch back, legs, thighs, bend to stretch hamstrings and back.

Tuesday, Thursday, Saturday

- 10-minute jog to get heart rate pumping.

- 20 reps calf raises x3 sets- flex feet lifting heels off the ground, flexes the calf muscle. For added resistance, carry a weight against your chest to mimic increased body weight.

- 1-minute jog in place to return heart rate to cardio level.

- 20 twist squats x3 sets- regular squat, twist to alternating sides to work glutes. Watch form and keep back straight to avoid overly twisting your back.

- Stair climb x3 reps- climb 1 flight of stairs in your home as quickly, yet safely as possible. If you only have one step, hop up and down alternating feet x 20 per rep.

- 30-second side plank x3 reps each side- for more, raise hips down toward the floor and back up instead of staying static.

- 1-minute jumping jacks to return heart rate to cardio level.

- Ab walk-out x10 reps- from standing position, bend and touch your toes. Walk hand out across floor until in a plank position, then back to original position.

- Stretch and cooldown- stretch back, legs, thighs, bend to stretch hamstrings and back.

Weeks 2-3: Double Week One

Very simply, we need to build stamina past our baseline. Take the workout from week one and double everything. The new routine should take about 1 hour. This can be done in two ways:

Variation 1:

10-minute jog, run through calisthenics portion once, followed by another 10-minute jog, then another round of calisthenics.

Variation 2:

20-minute jog followed by double sets of calisthenics.

To switch it up more, change the order in which you do the exercises. Just remember that maintaining cardio in between reps will help burn more fat while you complete your routine.

Weeks 4-5: Add in more targeted exercises

Use your baseline from week one to determine which muscle groups need more attention.

For example, if pull ups and arm workouts were toughest, put your focus there.

Depending on your commitment and availability of time, either add the following exercises into your circuit or trade them out for ones you have mastered.

Remember to keep up cardio in between.

This progression means you may need some extra equipment.

Invest in free weights or get creative around the house.

Empty milk or water gallon jugs filled with water or sand make great weights with handles.

Weights are adjustable by adding or subtracting water.

Keep several sets to mimic weights.

Use a home scale to determine weights or do it by feel.

Arm exercises

•	20 bicep curls x 3 reps: Use free weights or water jugs to create more resistance.

•	20 triceps kickback x3 reps using free weights or other heavy objects.

•	20 triceps extensions x3 reps.

Leg exercises

•	20 Scissor kicks x3 sets- lie on back and crisscross legs back and forth, also great for back and butt.

•	20 Plank leg lifts x3 sets- plank on hands, lift alternating legs as high as possible back and forth.

•	20 Squat sidekicks x3 sets- bend down to squat, when coming up, kick leg out to side as high as possible, alternate legs.

Core exercises

•	30-second wall sit x3 reps- for more, lift legs out one at a time for extra stretch.

•	30 sprinters x3 reps- from back, pull alternating legs to the chest while maintaining crunch position.

•	30 corkscrews x3 reps- from lying position, point legs up in the air, swirling them around the axis for a full stretch. For hip problems, simply raise and lower legs up and down vertically.

Weeks 6-7: Up the Cardio Intensity

Cardio is a big part of this equation.

By now, you should be used to a quick ten-minute interval jog.

Step it up a notch by alternating sprints.

Your ten minutes should include 3 one-minute sprints, running as fast as you can.

Your leg muscles should feel fatigued and shaky, that's how you know you're really working them out.

If you have more time, increase your total cardio time for added fat burning.

Also, increase the incline if possible.

Utilize stairs, incline on the treadmill or naturally occurring hills in your neighborhood.

Good news, this also counts as a great leg workout while getting that heart going.

Week 8: Revisit Baseline

Remember that strenuous exercise you did to determine your baseline?

If you tried and failed at a kickboxing class or CrossFit session, do it again.

Week 8 is all about measuring progress and setting up for another 8 weeks of workouts.

No routine is complete without a bit of tweaking as your baseline changes.

Use this week to redo week 1 and 2 exercises, complete your baseline challenge and prep for the weeks ahead.

If your baseline task is still very challenging, your workouts aren't doing enough for you.

Add more cardio if your heart still races, and add extra weights or reps if your muscles are failing you early on.

If your baseline task is now easy for you, congratulations!

You have reached your goal, and it is time to set a new one.

Try setting something more long term, like entering a strength and stamina competition, a triathlon or other competitive event.

If that's not your speed, try setting up a friendly challenge with people you know.

Getting others involved makes the process of working out fun, entertaining and social, three things that are a requirement for life-long program success.

You surely won't continue working out if you don't enjoy the new lifestyle changes.

Set up a new plan.

After week eight, you are free to use these exercises as you choose.

Create a fun and exciting workout with these movements, add some fresh new things and pair them with cardio exercises that are more stimulating than jogging.

The sky is the limit with exercise, so make it a goal to try some new things to keep it fresh.

Just remember to keep your ancient Greek friends in mind if you do.

Chapter 7: Proper Nutrition

Working out means nothing if you are not properly fueling your body.

Everywhere you look there is advice about proper eating techniques for your best body, and this book, too, will provide its own advice.

The difference here is that we will look at nutrition through the eyes of those we look to become, the ancient Greeks.

First, let's take a look at the science behind food.

It is important to know how different types of foods interact with our metabolism.

There are three major components of food; protein, carbohydrates and fat.

Each can be used for fuel in the body, as our metabolism is equipped to utilize anything available for survival.

As we discussed in the chapter on cardio exercise, simple sugars broken down from carbohydrates are the body's primary source of fuel.

The simple sugars that make up carbohydrates are not bound to other compounds and can chemically be broken down very quickly.

If the body was starved for fuel, carbohydrates can be utilized before the body expires.

In fact, carbohydrates serve no other purpose in the body except for energy.

These little nuggets of energy can be stored within the liver short term, or packed away and stored as fat for later use.

Because carbohydrates are so readily stored as fat, they should be limited in the diet.

Heavy carbs like potatoes and pasta should be limited or eliminated, while lower carb fruits should be chosen in their place.

Fruits also provide fiber, which cannot be broken down and used for energy, but helps keep the digestive tract moving.

Increased fiber keeps you full longer as it takes so much time to be broken down.

Protein from the diet is what muscle is made of, and will be the key ingredient to keeping muscles healthy and toned through your exercise regimen.

As muscles are worked, the fibers that make them fray and break, and must be repaired.

Protein from the diet is quickly shunted to muscles in need of repair to rebuild them quickly.

Proteins from the body are broken down into amino acids, which help build and repair muscles.

Protein can come from both plant and animal sources, however, animal proteins like chicken and fish provide a more complete amino acid profiles necessary for repair.

If you think about it, you are eating muscle from another animal to supplement and repair your own muscle.

Using plant proteins like soy will not give you the same variety of amino acids your muscles need to rebuild.

Dietary fat has a really bad reputation, one that is totally unwarranted.

Fat is a necessary nutrient to life and is absolutely essential to the function in our bodies.

It is responsible for cushioning our vital organs, works in cells to facilitate chemical reactions that drive life, and actually make up the majority of our brain mass.

We literally cannot think straight without fat.

Fats aid in the digestion of fat-soluble vitamins, help with hormone reactions, and a number of other supportive roles.

Yet, modern day diets have shunned fat, calling it the responsible party for weight gain.

Per gram, provides the most energy of the three macronutrients, and this is why the mob is after it.

A little bit of fat goes a long way, with just a teaspoon of olive oil carrying about one hundred calories.

In the past, it was thought that dietary fat was solely responsible for increasing fat stores in the body.

We now know that is untrue, as excess carbohydrates are more a culprit for fat storage than dietary fats.

Not all fats are created equal, and it is still necessary to use them sparingly because of their high-calorie content.

Small amounts of polyunsaturated fats, like olive oil and avocado keep the body running like a well-oiled machine.

Saturated animal fats like lard and butter should be eaten sparingly if at all, as they are transported through the blood in cholesterol.

Excess saturated fat increases cholesterol and blocks arteries causing heart disease.

Let's put this all together.

We now know that we need a variety of carbohydrates, protein and fats for a healthy body, despite what fad diets sling out for information.

The key is that we get them all in a balanced way.

In general, our plates should be balanced at every meal.

Focus half of your plate around non-starchy vegetables like salad, cooked broccoli, asparagus or tomato.

Potatoes and corn are considered starchy vegetables and should be considered a carbohydrate.

The other half of your plate should be split evenly between lean protein and carbohydrate.

Fats should be used sparingly, and consider them as a garnish.

If you like oil or have cooked the meat or vegetables in oil, stick to 1-2 teaspoonfuls per meal maximum, and make sure they are good quality oils like coconut, olive or avocado.

A common thread with bodybuilding is the use of excess protein to build muscles.

There are shelves full of products in health food stores that are loaded with amino acids for building muscles.

But what are the real benefits of that?

If you are a professional body builder in the business of growing massive muscles, extra protein will be required.

As we discussed earlier, breaking down muscles with exercise requires protein to build them back up.

Theoretically, if more protein is available, the muscle will prefer to bulk up with more fibers to be able to handle the extra weight next time.

This is simply physiology and is how to create stronger muscles.

Remember though, that our goal here isn't to create extreme muscles, it is to build upon the ones we have to make them more functional.

This doesn't require too much protein.

In fact, giving more protein than the muscles need will cause the excess to be converted and stored as fat.

Unless you are truly wearing out your muscles, excess protein means excess fat, and isn't that just a waste?

Instead, focus on getting the right amount of protein.

For the majority of healthy people, this equals out to 0.8grams of protein per kilogram body weight.

If you have some weight to lose, your protein needs will actually be a bit higher while you ration your portions down.

In general, if you are at your approximate goal weight, within ten to twenty pounds, use your actual body weight to determine your protein needs.

For example, a 180-pound man, 82 kilograms, will need about 66 grams of protein daily.

Exceeding this will only cause you to overstep your calorie needs for the day, leading to weight and fat gain.

If you are not sure how many calories you will need to maintain or lose weight, consult with your health care professional.

In general, it takes a deficit of 250 calories per day through diet and exercise to lose one pound per week, which is generally regarded as safe weight loss.

To determine what an appropriate weight is for your height, meet with your doctor or registered dietitian to set appropriate goals and get help with meal planning.

All of this is good advice, but how would the Greeks react to this meal pattern?

Honestly, it would probably follow their diets pretty closely.

The last century has brought so many bad things into our diets.

Advancements in food science allow foods to be preserved longer, but the preservatives are unnatural and make us sick.

Using things like high fructose corn syrup to make things taste sweeter has made once very enjoyable treats like fruit bitter and unappealing, leading the way for sugary drinks and snacks to make up the majority of our diets.

The typical American diet now consists of mostly carbohydrates, fat and salt, as this is what we have determined tastes good.

Unfortunately, these foods are high calorie and everything that our bodies do not need right away is stored as fat.

Not to mention the excess salt has our blood pressures through the roof.

Combine the overfeeding with under exercising and we have a recipe for obesity and disease, far from the Greek ideal we are setting out for.

Given that the world we live in is not conducive to a healthy lifestyle, we must look back to determine what worked well for our ancient Greek friends.

In that region during that time, there were only a few major food groups available.

First, there certainly were no processed foods, so they were automatically healthier.

The Greeks ate whatever they could forage or farm.

They had livestock which gave them milk and cheese.

They grew olives, a great healthy source of fat.

In summer months, they had an abundance of fresh fruits and vegetables, and for those who lived by the coast, endless supplies of seafood rich in healthy Omega 3 fatty acids.

They also cultivated grains, giving them bread and other cereal-based treats.

Most importantly, food was work.

These people did not just head to the grocery store to pick these things up.

They worked away on homestead farms, tending to livestock and crops on a daily basis.

An ounce of food was worth a day of work in those days, and everything was eaten in moderation to make it last.

Also, the Greeks did drink a bit of wine, so feel free to have some.

A glass a day has been proven to improve memory and cardiovascular health, just don't overdo it.

Take a note from ancient Greece and model your diet around what was available to them.

This will automatically eliminate a number of things that are contributing to the decline of health.

Eat whole, unprocessed foods from quality sources. Pick fresh fruits and vegetables, and high-quality lean meats.

Given this modern age, indulge in a few decadent treats here and there but if your goal is to look like a Greek warrior, you must act like them.

Chapter 8: Health Benefits of This Program

The goal of this diet is not just to have a great body, but to be healthier.

By following this diet and exercise advice, and striving to have a naturally lean and powerful body, you will be healthier than the majority of people out there.

Here, we are not striving to be bodybuilders, but to have bodies that can build things. There is a major difference.

People who use steroids and overwork their muscles for sheer size will not win out in the end.

Using artificial means to gain muscles that are good for nothing will not lead to good health.

Professional bodybuilders often leave good health in the dust for size, but do not often work on their cardiovascular health, or worry about how their kidneys are handling the supplements they take.

On the flip side, the idea of creating an ideal Greek body is all about good health the natural way.

Using proper diet and exercise techniques nurtures the body without creating extra stress.

Remember that bodybuilders often stress and tear their muscles, leaving their body in a constant state of repair.

While a bit of this is necessary, the body actually hates it.

Your immune system becomes heightened when it thinks it is under attack, and constant muscle repair indicates that you are fending for your life on the outside.

For your body's sake, pair moderate exercise with regular rest to make sure your body is comfortable and stress-free.

If your immune system is taxed, it means it is not taking care of infections and disease that is floating around your body like it should.

While that body builder seems healthy now, their health will likely take a turn if they continue burning both ends of the candle.

In order to reap the health benefits of ancient Greeks, you must truly embrace the lifestyle.

Greek gods and warriors lived in a much different time.

They lived in an era before modern conveniences and were a much busier people.

There was no time to sit around, and really no reason to as television, video games and computers had yet to be invented.

Instead, these people were active in their communities, out enjoying nature, and for a select few, training to become Greek warriors.

Should you embrace the Greek lifestyle and live with the purpose of creating a body that is both healthy and functional, you will reap the benefits, and they should be obvious.

First, you will likely get the body you always dreamed of, which is probably what attracted you to this book.

Working out and fueling your body only with what it needs will lead to great muscle tone and decreased fat.

You will look great at the beach and your friends will wonder how you did it.

The health benefits of a trimmer body are also a great reason to get started.

Having a body that is within a normal weight for your height will decrease your risk of all sorts of health problems.

Obesity is associated with heart disease, diabetes, cancer and a host of other problems as weight increases.

Being in better health overall slows the aging process by creating less stress on your entire body, especially your heart and joints.

Eating better, a major component of this program will also ensure that your body stays in tip top shape.

Limiting bad fats that lead to plaque buildup and heart attacks is a major benefit of this plan.

Also, avoiding processed foods means avoiding chemical fillers that tax the liver and kidneys, and have the potential to cause cancer.

Regular exercise, especially those targeted toward increasing functional strength and cardiovascular stamina mean a healthier heart and lung system as you age.

Starting off strong now means less likelihood of steep decline, and starting from a better point of function improves your overall survival into older age.

Good nutrition and exercise also boost your immune system, giving you the ability to fight off infection.

Besides the physical health benefits, we must also look at mental health.

Studies in recent decades have shown that regular exercise and a great diet keep your brain healthy and decrease the chances of having mental health issues like anxiety, depression or other mood disorders.

The combination of healthy fats and flow of oxygen, among other things, keeps the brain fresh and active.

Being in better health overall can help you socially and financially as well.

Being in better shape means you will likely feel more confident about yourself, leading to more social interaction.

Those who have better social skills say they have a better overall quality of life and a better support system.

Being more social may also mean making the connections necessary to further your career.

Networking is key to being successful at any job.

Yes, you may be good at your job, but do you have the confidence to show it off?

If not, it is time to get your physical and mental health in order to make sure you get noticed.

Make a positive step in your life by committing just eight weeks to trying the Greek lifestyle.

Use the exercise regimen and diet advice to transform yourself physically and mentally.

Getting healthier, despite specific Golden Rule measurements will improve your life dramatically.

Reap the health benefits by making this advice part of your overall lifestyle.

Live a better quality of life by being more active and present in your daily activities.

Conclusion

Thanks for making it through to the end of *Bodybuilding: How to Build the Body of a Greek God.*

This text has been about much more than creating the body of a Greek god.

We must remember that to be a god we must exude confidence and power.

Yes, this begins with confidence in a physical capacity, but also transcends into many other aspects of our lives.

We cannot overlook the overall lifestyle that Greek warriors led in order to achieve these ideal bodies.

They were active members of society, and used brute strength and stamina on a daily basis, chiseling their bodies without even trying.

This was followed up with a healthy diet of foods they grew and raised themselves, putting in energy that is not necessary with our modern conveniences today.

Let's hope it was informative and able to provide you with all of the tools you need to achieve your goals of living like a Greek god.

If you hope to have the body of a Greek god, you must learn to adjust your lifestyle to one which supports the maintenance of this body.

Surely, the exercise program outlined in this book will set you well on your way, but eating like a modern American and sitting for the majority of the day will not give you lasting results.

Make some positive changes that will make it easy and sustainable to have a great body, rather than forcing it into an otherwise lethargic and gluttonous lifestyle.

The Greeks were truly healthier beings, and that should be the point to strive for. A rocking body is just a bonus.

Finally, if you found this book useful in any way, a review on Amazon is always appreciated!